Play, Playfulness, Creativity and Innovation

What roles do playful behaviour and playful thought take in animal and human development? How does play relate to creativity and, in turn, to innovation?

Unravelling the different meanings of 'play', this book focuses on non-aggressive playful play. The authors emphasise its significance for development and evolution, before examining the importance of playfulness in creativity. This discussion sheds new light on the links between creativity and innovation, distinguishing between the generation of novel behaviour and ideas on the one hand, and the implementation of these novelties on the other. The authors then turn to the role of play in the development of the child and to parallels among play, humour and dreaming, along with the altered states of consciousness generated by some psychoactive drugs. A final chapter looks ahead to future research and to what remains to be discovered in this fascinating and important field.

PATRICK BATESON FRS is Emeritus Professor of Ethology at the University of Cambridge. He is President of the Zoological Society of London and a former Vice-President of the Royal Society. Much of his scientific career has been concerned with the development of behaviour. He is also co-author of *Plasticity, Robustness, Development and Evolution* (Cambridge, 2011).

PAUL MARTIN studied behavioural biology at the University of Cambridge before becoming a Harkness Fellow in the Department of Psychiatry and Behavioral Sciences at Stanford University. He has lectured and researched in behavioural biology at the University of Cambridge and is a former Fellow of Wolfson College.

The authors have published other successful books together, including *Measuring Behaviour: An Introductory Guide* (3rd edition, Cambridge, 2007).

Play, Playfulness, Creativity and Innovation

PATRICK BATESON

and

PAUL MARTIN

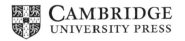

CAMBRIDGE
UNIVERSITY PRESS

University Printing House, Cambridge CB2 8BS, United Kingdom

Published in the United States of America by Cambridge University Press, New York

Cambridge University Press is part of the University of Cambridge.

It furthers the University's mission by disseminating knowledge in the pursuit of education, learning and research at the highest international levels of excellence.

www.cambridge.org
Information on this title: www.cambridge.org/9781107015135

© P. Bateson and P. Martin 2013

First published 2013

Printed in the United Kingdom by Clays, St Ives plc

A catalogue record for this publication is available from the British Library

Library of Congress Cataloguing in Publication data
Bateson, P. P. G. (Paul Patrick Gordon), 1938–
Play, playfulness, creativity and innovation / Patrick Bateson,
University of Cambridge and Paul Martin, Wolfson College, Cambridge.
    pages   cm.
ISBN 978-1-107-01513-5 (hardback)
1. Play – Psychological aspects.   2. Creative ability.   3. Creative
thinking.   I. Martin, Paul H., 1958–   II. Title.
BF717.B28   2013
155–dc23

                                              2013001078

ISBN 978-1-107-01513-5 Hardback
ISBN 978-1-107-68934-3 Paperback

Additional resources for this publication at www.cambridge.org/9781107015135

Contents

Advance praise

"This groundbreaking work will inform, engage and please an extensive audience, from play scholars and naturalists to those seeking an improved basis for practical approaches to social questions. The book's originality, common-sense foundation, clear and readable language, and pragmatism are all commendable. The authors, whose landmark studies of behavioral development now span more than a quarter century, take pains to present a readable and direct exposition of their ideas. At the same time, they succeed in drawing bold distinctions when necessary and in forthrightly addressing concerns that span a broad range of social issues.

The authors informatively fine-tune previous concepts of play in their successful efforts to link play with the origins of the creative process across a broad biological spectrum. The book's main themes – play as a driver of creative developmental options, play as a source of behavioral novelty to be integrated in the behavioral and social repertoire through the separate process of innovation, and play as a source of ideas and approaches for addressing broader issues of individuality and society – are woven together to produce a work of great general interest."

– Robert M. Fagen, author of *Animal Play Behavior*

"Play will be to the 21st century what work was to the industrial age – our dominant way of knowing, doing and creating value. Therefore we need play theory and research, of a multidisciplinary and consilient nature, that can deepen and widen our understanding of this most dynamic of our human evolved capacities – so that we can design the best games and technologies, communities and organisations, that will constitute this new era. Patrick Bateson and Paul Martin have provided here a wonderful resource for play/game advocates in all fields of life. Rooted in extremely solid biological and ethological research, they make subtle and powerful linkages between the mammalian basis of play, and the necessary profusion of social and cultural forms it generates, in ways that will help shape reform in areas as diverse as childcare, innovative enterprise and even drugs policy. *Play, Playfulness, Creativity and Innovation* sets a new standard for studies of the power and potential of play."

– **Pat Kane**, musician and author of *The Play Ethic*

"Kittens toy with half-dead prey, dogs chase sticks, kids pretend to be teachers or airline pilots, and their parents revel in painting, gardening and sport. All are examples of play behavior. But whilst it is immediately apparent that play is gratifying, a compelling scientific explanation for why it evolved in the first place has remained elusive. Now Bateson and Martin, leading experts on animal behavior, provide an answer – play functions to generate creativity and stimulate innovation. It is an adaptation to get out of the rut and discover better solutions to life's challenges. With beautifully clear writing and covering diverse literatures, from animal cognition, to child development, to dreaming and psychedelic drugs, Bateson and Martin's text provides a wonderfully readable and much-needed summary of scientific knowledge of play."

– **Kevin N. Laland**, University of St Andrews

"An important book at an important time. Yet again we are arguing over how best to fit our children to become useful productive citizens. Yes, we want them to be happy too, but the framework must somehow be put in. Play may be seen as a nice extra, part of becoming socially integrated. Bateson and Martin argue it is much, much more. Reviewing a wide range of studies, beginning with play in some of our animal relatives then to ourselves from infancy to adult life, with individuals and with businesses or institutions, they show how playfulness may be at the very core of creative thinking and action. During play we experiment, thinking outside the box, as we say. What can be established is a flexible framework much more adaptable to changing circumstances.

In effect, this book celebrates the human free spirit and is full of encouraging examples of what can be achieved. I hope it is widely studied in educational circles. Here some rich parents compete for tutors to get their 3 year olds into 'good' nursery schools and hence a 'good' primary at 5. In Finland, which out-scores us on most educational outcomes, primary begins at 7; two or three more years of play perhaps?"

– **Aubrey Manning**, University of Edinburgh, co-author of
An Introduction to Animal Behaviour (Cambridge, 6th edition, 2012)

"In this highly readable and thought-provoking book, Patrick Bateson and Paul Martin show how play helps animals to find novel solutions and sows the evolutionary seeds for human creativity. They argue that being able to 'break the rules' in a protected environment, which is what play does, generates new ideas (creativity) and new ways of doing things (innovation). By looking at the conditions in which humans are at their most creative, they make a major contribution to what we might do to be even more creative than we are."

– **Marian Stamp Dawkins**, University of Oxford, co-author of
An Introduction to Animal Behaviour (Cambridge, 6th edition, 2012)

Preface

This book had its origins in the early 1980s, when we were working together at Cambridge University's Sub-Department of Animal Behaviour on the developmental origins of behaviour. Our research led us to become increasingly interested in play behaviour and its role in enabling the developing organism to acquire valuable skills and experience. We promised ourselves that one day we would write a book together on the subject. However, we were also preoccupied with many other duties. Work on the present book was put off again and again, although we collaborated on two other books, one of which is now in its third edition (Bateson & Martin, 1999; Martin & Bateson, 2007). Finally, though, we started to develop our ideas about play in book form.

The different meanings given to the term 'play' have created much confusion and have contributed to the view that play is enigmatic and almost beyond the boundaries of science. The categorisation of play as any behaviour that is not 'serious' has tended to trivialise an activity that is likely to have important beneficial outcomes, both in humans and other species. We became particularly interested in the links between playfulness and creativity, and aware of the difference between generating novel forms of behaviour or ideas (creativity) and implementing worthwhile inventions in a practical way (innovation). Inevitably the book has taken on a different shape from what we had originally envisaged and the focus has enlarged to take in other aspects of human affairs. Playful play can be a serious business.

One reader of an early draft version complained about our cautious use of phrases like 'may be important' and so forth, as though we were not quite confident enough to make the big points without qualifying them. We accept that this book is academic in its approach, and that where the evidence is equivocal or absent, we have said so. The book is aimed in part at academic biologists and psychologists. Our emphasis is on empirical evidence and on where further research needs to be carried out because the evidence is incomplete. However, we hope that our conclusions will also interest those who are concerned with creativity and innovation, whether for the public good or for commercial benefit. Playfulness in adult life affects the readiness with which people develop new ideas and has a broad influence on human relations. Given the importance of play in child development, we hope too that those involved in education will read it.

Patrick Bateson
Paul Martin
November 2012

Acknowledgements

We are very grateful to a number of friends and colleagues who read the drafts of the whole book. They are: Teresa Belton, Robert Fagen, Emma Flynn, Kevin Laland, Eugene Lim, Corina Logan and Aubrey Manning. We thank them and the following who read parts of the book in draft: Max Alexander, Jacqueline Barnes, Anna Bateson, Zahaan Bharmal, Nick Humphrey, Ben Malbon, Harriet Martin and Daniel Nettle. It goes without saying that they all contributed to the final version in a variety of invaluable ways and that all sins of omission and commission are our own. For part of the project, P.B. received a grant for his research from the Leverhulme Trust, which he thanks for its support.

1

Introduction

This book is about the role of play and playfulness in creativity and innovation. We argue that play is an important form of behaviour that facilitates creativity, and hence innovation, in both the natural world and human society. Although the consequences of play are most obvious during the lifetime of each individual, play also affects biological evolution by enabling organisms to adapt rapidly to novel environments.

The essence of our argument is that playful behaviour and playful thought can generate radically new approaches to challenges set by the physical and social environment. While our approach grew out of observations of non-human animals by biologists, we argue that humans and organisations can exploit playfulness as a tool for fostering creativity and innovation.

'Play' evidently has many different meanings, some of which refer to aspects of behaviour and thinking that are very different from the playful mode of behaviour on which we shall focus. For example, rule-governed competitive sports are 'played', but they are rarely conducted playfully. Sports and many games are often treated as being deadly serious. Similarly, theatrical plays in which the actors are required to have learned their lines are not associated with the lightness of mood which we regard as being so important in playful creativity. Stage improvisation and ad libbing, however, may come closer to what we have in mind.

PLAYFULNESS

Apart from its many different colloquial usages, 'play' – as used by biologists and psychologists – is a broad term denoting almost any activity that is not 'serious' or 'work'. Play may also be defined more specifically, according to several criteria:

- the behaviour is spontaneous and rewarding to the individual
- it is intrinsically motivated and its performance is a goal in itself
- the behaviour occurs in a protected context when the player is neither ill nor stressed
- the behaviour is incomplete or exaggerated relative to non-playful behaviour in adults
- it is performed repeatedly.

While play is often regarded principally as an activity of young animals or children, it also occurs in adults of many species.

Part of our thesis in this book rests on the distinction we have drawn between observable play behaviour and an underlying mood state that we refer to as playfulness. Play behaviour may or may not be playful. 'Playfulness' is a particular positive mood state that may (or may not) be manifested in observable behaviour. Playfulness facilitates and accompanies 'playful play', a subset of broadly defined play, which is distinct from what happens in formal games, theatrical performances and so forth. Play and playfulness do overlap, but we believe the distinction is important because some aspects of play behaviour are not playful, particularly when they start to merge into overt competition or aggression. Aspects of what many biologists and psychologists would subsume under the general heading of 'play' may be driven by frustration or striving for social dominance. An encounter that starts off in a way that is described as playful may degenerate into overt aggression, when the lightness of mood associated with other aspects of play seems to be lacking. Conversely, playful individuals are not necessarily playing, even though they are in a playful mood. We shall consider in greater detail how play and playfulness are characterised in Chapter 2.

The notion of 'playful play' is our own and is not to be found in the academic literature. We suggest that this new category helps in the understanding of a motivational state that is important in creativity. Our restrictive use of the term is captured in Figure 1.1, which shows the incomplete overlap between this aspect of play and other aspects encompassed by less restrictive but widely accepted definitions of play. Both these domains overlap with an even larger one in which the loosest definitions of 'play' are more extensive and the variety of meanings is evident.

We recognise that play continues to be something of an enigma and much more needs to be discovered. In our final chapter we outline some of the many questions that remain to be answered through empirical research. Until they have a firmer basis in evidence, some of the widely believed theories about play must remain in the realm of conjecture.

CREATIVITY AND INNOVATION

In this book we draw a simple distinction between creativity and innovation. In human behaviour, creativity refers broadly to generating new ideas, whereas innovation refers to changing the way in which things are done. Although creativity and innovation are often treated as synonymous (e.g. Feist, 1998), we believe the terms can usefully be distinguished. Creativity is displayed when an individual develops a novel form of behaviour or a novel idea, regardless of its practical uptake and subsequent application. Innovation means implementing a novel form of behaviour or an idea in order to obtain a practical benefit which is then adopted by others. As Max Mckeown (2008) succinctly put it: 'Innovation is new stuff that is made useful'. In many of the human examples that we consider later, creative people are not necessarily innovative, and innovative people may rely on the novel ideas or actions of other more creative people.

The distinction between creativity and innovation is harder to observe in other species. Even so, animals can be

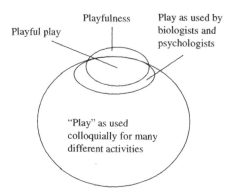

Figure 1.1. The relationship between playfulness and play as commonly described by biologists and psychologists. These overlap with the many different colloquial usages of 'play' for competitive games, theatrical events and so forth.

creative and they do innovate; for example, by discovering new ways of obtaining food. Considerable time can elapse between a creative act by one individual and a subsequent innovation in which other individuals adopt the new way of doing things. What is observed is often the end product of a long process.

THE THESIS

The core of our argument is that new forms of behaviour and new modes of thought frequently derive from play, and especially from playful play. Such activity is a driver of creativity and, less directly, of innovation, both in humans and in other species. Play generates novel ways of dealing with the environment, most of which lead nowhere but some of which turn out to be useful.

Much of animal and human behaviour involves trade-offs between conflicting requirements. In making those trade-offs, the individual may be trapped on the metaphorical equivalent of a false mountain summit – what engineers call a local optimum – with a higher peak beyond. When that happens, the individual needs a way of getting off the lower peak in order to discover the most satisfactory solution – the global optimum.

We shall argue that play is an evolved biological adaptation that enables the individual to escape from local optima and discover better solutions.

The concept of play applies to thoughts as well as visible actions. Humans can think playfully as well as act playfully, generating novel patterns of thought in a protected context. A large part of human play goes on in the mind and may not manifest itself in overt behaviour. When play is overt, it may be seen more often in children than in adults, but adult humans are perfectly capable of playing and, we shall argue, sometimes benefit from it. As George Bernard Shaw remarked: 'We don't stop playing because we grow old, we grow old because we stop playing'.

Play enables the individual to discover new approaches to dealing with the world. We distinguish this, as others have done, from exploration, whereby the individual systematically gathers new information about the world. Typically, exploratory behaviour in animals begins cautiously and, as the individual gathers confidence, becomes both more extensive and more intense. It is not immediately repeated unless the previously explored features of the environment change (Fagen, 1981). Play behaviour, on the other hand, is generally far from cautious: it is typically repeated many times and its very exuberance often leads the player into blind alleys. Who cares about blind alleys when you are having fun? But even though play and exploration are substantially different, they are not entirely unrelated, and humans may sometimes be regarded as exploring playfully.

A notable characteristic of play behaviour is that it generally does not appear to have an immediate practical goal or benefit. Indeed, some writers implicitly define play as anything that seems pointless. Play appears to provide its own reward, at least in the short term, by being intrinsically enjoyable. The general presumption has been that the more tangible biological benefits of play usually come later in the individual's lifetime; for example, in the form of improved physical, cognitive or social skills. The gap in time between playing and making use of the experience acquired during play may be measured in months or even years.

This temporal disjunction between experience and later performance has proved important in interpreting apparently insightful solutions to problems, when the individual seemingly plumps instantly for the right answer without testing the alternatives. The experience that enabled it to respond promptly to the new challenge occurred earlier in its life, when playing. We discuss this important aspect of experience gained through play in Chapters 5 and 6. Even though a time gap often occurs between play experience and beneficial outcomes, the effect of play may in some cases be immediate. In such cases, the individual acquires skills that increase its current chances of survival or it solves a problem, with immediate benefit.

Among the biological benefits of play, we contend, are creativity and innovation. In Chapter 7 we discuss how play and playfulness may boost the creativity of adult humans, both as individuals and collectively through the activities of organisations. In Chapter 8 we consider the evidence that children's creativity can be enhanced by play. Playfulness in humans is often associated with humour, and we discuss this relationship in Chapter 9. States of consciousness that are different from the normal waking state are obvious enough in dreaming and daydreaming. The dreaming or daydreaming individual may be generating novel patterns of thought and, in some senses, does this in a protected context. Both are features of play. We discuss the parallels between play and altered states of consciousness in Chapter 10, and go on to consider how some drug-induced states can be associated with enhanced creativity. Finally, in Chapter 11, we attempt to pull the threads together and offer suggestions for future research.

HISTORY

Before going further, it is worth considering briefly the long history of debate over the nature of play and its role in the development of individual humans. The role of play in the education of children has engaged numerous writers from a variety of backgrounds over many centuries. Plato, writing some 2,400 years ago in *The Laws*, argued that playful practice when young is important for the development of adult skills. Jean-Jacques Rousseau (1712–78) thought that play in a natural environment civilises the child. The philosopher Immanuel Kant (1724–1804) took a romantic view of play as liberating the spirit. So too did the poet Friedrich Schiller (1759–1805), who believed that play allows the release of pent-up energy. The psychologist Karl Groos (1861–1946) argued, like Plato, that adult skills are acquired during childhood play. The educational reformer John Dewey (1859–1952) was influenced by Rousseau and regarded play as crucially important in the development of the child. Sigmund Freud (1856–1939) wrote about its importance to an individual's subsequent behaviour, and many other psychoanalysts and psychotherapists have followed in his footsteps (e.g. Erikson, 1963). None of these authors explicitly linked play to creativity. Herbert Spencer did, however, and suggested that play is the source of artistic creativity (Spencer, 1872).

The historian Johan Huizinga (1955), taking a very broad view of play, argued that it is important in the development of all aspects of human culture. As he put it: 'Genuine, pure play is one of the main bases of civilisation'. The Russian psychologist Lev Vygotsky (1967), writing in the 1930s, took a more specific view: he believed that literacy and imagination derive from the actions involved in play. Another influential developmental psychologist, Jean Piaget (1952), initially believed that play is important for the development of a logical mind, but in a later book argued that play is important in the development of the child's imagination (Piaget, 1962). In more recent times, scholarly writing on play has proliferated.[1]

Some writers, taking a similar line to Vygotsky, have argued that play is the precursor of imaginative writing (e.g. Smith, 1982). Brian Sutton-Smith (1986) suggested that the foundations for an aptitude for imaginative writing are established in babyhood when babies and their mothers play 'face games' with each other and, through incongruity, joy and laughter, establish the basis for expressive performances. He concluded, though without citing any empirical evidence: 'This is the most probable source of both later symbolic play and later story-telling'. In a more sceptical vein than in his earlier work, Sutton-Smith (1997) noted that while various theories disagree about the specific kinds of development instigated by play, they all assume that play experience does indeed transfer to other activities that are not in themselves forms of play. Sutton-Smith did use the term 'play' very broadly to cover many serious activities, and we suspect that much of what he referred to as 'the ambiguity of play' stems from the multifaceted use of the word and not the more specific sense in which we use it here.

An important milestone in the development of a scientific approach to play was Robert Fagen's (1981) book *Animal Play Behavior*. Fagen adopted an evolutionary approach and raised the question of why birds and mammals should spend time and energy on play, incurring risks as they do so. A number of other important books on play have appeared more recently.[2] None, however, has explored at length the link between playfulness and creativity.

CONCLUSIONS

Apart from its multifaceted usages, 'play' is a broad term denoting any activity that is not 'serious' or 'work' and is therefore generally associated with childhood rather than adult life. Biologists typically define play more specifically as intrinsically rewarding behaviour that occurs in a protected context in which players are largely insulated from the consequences of their behaviour, and uses behaviour patterns in unusual forms or combinations. The biological concept of play applies to thoughts as well as physical actions. 'Playfulness' is a positive mood state that facilitates and accompanies 'playful play', a subset of broadly defined play. Our thesis is that play, and especially playful play, facilitates creativity – sometimes immediately and sometimes after a considerable delay. We distinguish creativity, the generation of novel actions or thoughts, from innovation, in which new ways of doing things are implemented and adopted by others.

2

The biology of play

The definition of play has been a recurrent bugbear in the biological literature, as Robert Fagen (1981) recognised in his groundbreaking book *Animal Play Behavior*. Part of the problem is that human observers are all too ready to interpret other species' behaviour in terms of their own experience. Their definitions are ostensive rather than operational – that is to say, they point to a real example of the behaviour and say: 'That is what we mean by play'. For those scientists who are not present to be shown what is meant, the definition may be supported by verbal descriptions, drawings or videos. Such descriptions of play are often accompanied by the statement that the behaviour is not serious, in the sense that it does not apparently satisfy an immediate biological need of the individual, such as obtaining food or winning a fight.

The label 'play', when applied to animal behaviour, draws attention to how readily humans project onto other animals the perceptions they have of themselves and their fellow human beings. Such projection was revealed in many people's reactions to a beautifully illustrated book called *Why Cats Paint* by Busch and Silver (1994), which caused a flurry of interest among art critics. The book contained paintings supposedly produced by cats. Like those by some captive chimpanzees, the cats' artistic creations were seen as 'joyous and full of life'. Moreover, the cats were not simply creating abstract pictures, they were said to be doing so playfully. The book attracted serious reviews in major newspapers, amazing though this may seem. The reviewers had apparently failed to notice the list of references at the back of the book, which included telltale entries such as this:

Lord-osis, J. (1991) Pawnography: Paw marking as a mode of sexual communication among domestic cats in Sweden. *J. Appl. Aesthetics*, Vol VI.

The whole book was, of course, a spoof. It demonstrated (playfully) how easily humans, scientists included, fall into the trap of supposing that animals are like us. This is not to deny the growing body of scientific opinion that most, if not all, vertebrates are conscious and aware of their surroundings and experiences (Bekoff, 2010). Nevertheless, considerable care must be applied when articulating categories of behaviour observed in other species. Establishing such categories provides the basis for the measurement that is a crucial part of behavioural biology.

In the case of play, scepticism about the distinctiveness of this category is often shrugged off because, it is claimed, everybody recognises play when they see it. However, recognition is not the same as agreement. When a kitten plays, observers will readily agree about its activities and their quantified measurements will correlate strongly with each other (Caro et al., 1979). But when a fish does something that might be called play, many scientists will remain sceptical about whether it is really playing (e.g. Manning & Dawkins, 2012). The subtle attributions that accompany the naming of behavioural categories in animals have to be watched carefully. This care should be extended to the way that children's behaviour is categorised by adult humans. Using a term like 'play' to describe a child's behaviour may imply an understanding of the child's motivation that goes beyond the actual evidence. Such an assumption may lead to the conclusion that everything a child does without obvious need is play. In our view, play and playfulness are more specific categories with other defining characteristics.

DEFINING PLAY

Over the years a number of psychologists and biologists have attempted to bring order to the subject of play by listing the various criteria by which play behaviour might be recognised (e.g. Burghardt, 2005; Fagen, 1981). Five defining features of play, which have emerged from studies of play in many species, are central to our thesis. They are as follows.

1. The behaviour is spontaneous and rewarding to the individual; it is intrinsically motivated and its performance serves as a goal in itself. Play is 'fun'.

2. The player is to some extent protected from the normal consequences of serious behaviour. The behaviour appears to have no immediate practical goal or benefit. Social forms of the behaviour may be preceded or accompanied by specific signals or facial expressions indicating that the behaviour is not serious. Play is the antithesis of 'work' or 'serious' behaviour.

3. The behaviour consists of actions or, in the case of humans, thoughts, expressed in novel combinations. Social forms of the behaviour may be accompanied by temporary changes in social relationships, such as role reversals, in which a normally dominant individual may become temporarily subordinate while playing, and vice versa. Play is a generator of novelty.

4. Individual actions or thoughts are performed repeatedly (though they do not resemble stereotypies such as the circular pacing seen in animals kept in deprived conditions); they may also be incomplete or exaggerated relative to non-playful behaviour in adults. Play looks different.

5. The behaviour is sensitive to prevailing conditions and occurs only when the player is free from illness or stress. Play is an indicator of well-being.

These criteria overlap extensively with those articulated by Gordon Burghardt (2005), who devoted a substantial portion of his book to characterising the defining features of play and relating them to observational evidence from numerous species.[3] His analysis led him to suggest five criteria by which play can be recognised. They are broadly similar to the core features listed above, though we do have some quibbles. Burghardt insisted that all five criteria should apply if an animal is said to be playing. This may make application difficult, since obtaining evidence about function and the animal's internal state are problematical. One of his criteria applies primarily to social behaviour and is not a core feature of object play. Moreover,

Burghardt relaxed the criteria when considering the precursors of play in vertebrates other than birds and mammals, and in some invertebrates.

The five criteria listed above define play in the sense in which many biologists and psychologists use the term, and how we use it in this book. But they do not define *playful* play. For play to be playful, a sixth feature must also be present:

6.   Playful play (as distinct from the broader biological category of play) is accompanied by a particular positive mood state in which the individual is more inclined to behave (and, in the case of humans, think) in a spontaneous and flexible way.

We have drawn a distinction between playful play and non-playful play. Playfulness, the defining feature of playful play, is a positive mood state that is not always detectable in observable behaviour. The behaviour of a playful human is captured by numerous synonyms, including cheerful, frisky, frolicsome, good-natured, joyous, merry, rollicking, spirited, sprightly and vivacious. Some of these terms relate to human emotions that could not be readily identified in animals without much anthropomorphic projection. Some, though, are descriptive of visible behaviour and can be defined ostensively, such as when kittens engage vigorously in social play. In animals, as in humans, playfulness may be inferred from the context in which it occurs. What the animals do may vary – from playing with objects at one moment to playing with another individual at the next – but the playful state underlying their behaviour is the same.

PLAY IN HUMANS

Play, as defined above, can manifest itself in many different ways in humans. It may be solitary, social, pretend, imaginary, symbolic, verbal, socio-dramatic, constructional, rough-and-tumble, manipulative, and so forth (Pellegrini, 2009; Power, 2000). These different forms of play differ in their structure, their underlying motivation and, quite probably, their biological functions. For example, the rough-and-tumble play of a 4-year-old child wrestling with another 4-year-old is visibly very different from that of, say, a solitary 10-year-old staring into space, lost in a fantasy. The criteria for recognising play in animals work well when applied to the rough-and-tumble play of a child, but pretend play requires additional definition (Mitchell, 2007; Smith, 2010). Applying non-literal meanings to actions and objects is a central feature of pretend play in humans. It involves imitative actions in a non-functional context, such as pressing a toy stethoscope against the chest of a doll.

Such instances of pretend play are easy to define by pointing to examples, and a case can be made for defining similar behaviour seen in the great apes. For example, young female chimpanzees behave maternally towards sticks, ceasing to do so when they have real offspring to care for (Kahlenberg & Wrangham, 2010). This stick-carrying behaviour consists of holding or cradling sticks, pieces of bark, small logs or woody vines with the hand or mouth, underarm or, most commonly, tucked between the abdomen and thigh. Individuals carry sticks for periods ranging from a minute to more than 4 hours, during which time they rest, walk, climb, sleep and feed as usual. The occurrence of stick-carrying is greatest among juvenile females and resembles the pretend play of human children.

The pretend play of older children, who can describe what they are thinking and doing, may be viewed as part of a package of characteristically human behaviour and cognition, much of which is internalised. This complex package includes the use of language, self-awareness, and an understanding of how other humans think and are likely to behave (Smith, 2010). The definition we have used above would not readily apply to such examples, although many could be described as playful.

We should emphasise an important point contained in the core features listed above – namely, that the concept of play applies to thoughts as well as to overt physical actions. Humans can play in the realm of pure thought and their play can generate creative solutions to problems. We return to this theme later when considering altered states of consciousness, such as dreaming, and their relationship with play and creativity.

BAD PLAY

Our criteria for recognising play would exclude behaviour in which the player is stressed or hurt by another. In reporting their own experiences, some authors have described how frightening rough-and-tumble play can be and the humiliation of, say, being pinned to the ground by a bigger child. These unpleasant aspects of human 'play' can include teasing, bullying, shunning, hurting and being hurt. For instance, Robin Henig (2008) wrote: 'I well remember this darker side of play from my own girlhood ... I had to wait to be asked to play jump-rope and had to face embarrassment if I missed a skip or – worse, much worse – if nobody ended up asking me. Even pretend play could take an ugly turn if my playmates made their dolls say nasty things.'

The negative side of 'play' is also apparent in other animals. For example, researchers observed how male adult horses who were most likely to initiate what looked like play were also the ones who, according to other criteria, were the most chronically stressed. The stressed horses behaved as though the 'play' were an outlet for frustrated aggression (Hausberger et al., 2012). If so, this would not constitute play in the terms that we listed earlier, and it would certainly not be playful play. Similarly, Bateson (2011) noticed how tense kittens could be just before launching themselves at a sibling. They would arch their backs and swish their tails. If grabbed from behind by a human during that preparatory phase, they would scream, apparently in fright, and retreat from the other individual. They lacked the positive, relaxed mood associated with playfulness, but if they had not been disturbed, their mood would have relaxed and their behaviour would have satisfied the core features we identified. Mood can also change in the opposite direction. Occasionally, social play degenerates into a spat and the behaviour becomes aggressive. For one of the participating individuals, the encounter can become disagreeable and the playful mood rapidly evaporates. Although some writers continue to describe the behaviour in such encounters as play, we think the change of mood means that the behaviour can no longer be regarded as playful, and if the individual becomes stressed then it may no longer even constitute play.

PLAY ACROSS THE ANIMAL KINGDOM

Play behaviour has been recognised in a large number of mammal and bird species. As far as the behaviour of young mammals is concerned, it seems likely that few, if any, species will be found where play in one form or another is absent. In birds, play has been recorded in parrots, hornbills, babblers and members of the crow family (Diamond & Bond, 2003). The existence or not of play in other vertebrate taxonomic groups is much more controversial (Manning & Dawkins, 2012). Gordon Burghardt (2005) examined the possibility of play in taxonomic groups other than birds and mammals. He identified instances of behaviour in fish and reptiles that looked rather like object play in birds and mammals. According to Burghardt, some invertebrates – such as octopus and even spiders – might also exhibit play-like behaviour. For example, sexual acts between males and immature female spiders that do not result in the union of sperm and egg are found to decrease the subsequent latency to an act resulting in fertilisation and to increase maternal investment in the offspring (Pruitt & Riechert, 2011). In a subsequent paper, Pruitt, Burghardt and Riechert (2012) argued that the non-conceptive behaviour had formal similarities with play in birds and mammals. The conclusion that spiders and other invertebrates engage in play may seem implausible, even if it does follow logically from a precise definition that works for birds and mammals. What this example illustrates is the considerable difficulty in defining play.

HETEROGENEOUS CATEGORIES

As in humans, the play of other species can manifest itself in distinctly different forms. For example, when describing play in a mammal as generally playful as the domestic cat, it becomes clear that different components of its play behaviour are displayed in different situations. For instance, arching of the back, which is often seen in social play, does not appear in play with objects (Barrett & Bateson, 1978). Similarly, pouncing on objects, especially furry objects, is not seen in locomotor play (Egan, 1976; Martin & Bateson, 1985). Moreover, the developmental trajectories of these different forms of play are not the same. In cats, social play starts well before weaning, whereas object play increases sharply in the seventh week after birth, several weeks after the kittens have started to take solid food (Barrett & Bateson, 1978). Different structural features are therefore required to characterise these different subcategories of play.

Dolphins are magnificently playful animals and particularly good subjects for investigating the different manifestations of play. Captive dolphins play readily with balls and other toys. In the wild, they play with feathers, seaweed, sponges and other objects. They also play with bubble rings, which they create for themselves from their blowholes. Dolphins play with these items in a variety of ways, such as pushing them around, throwing them in the air, or swimming through their bubble rings. They are also highly social, playing extensively with each other. Thirty-seven different types of play have been described in the young of the bottlenose dolphin (Kuczaj et al., 2006). Examples include holding a ball, swimming and tossing a ball simultaneously, using the mouth or chin to dribble a ball at the surface or under the water, pushing a ball with a body part, trapping a ball between a hard surface and part of the body, using a ball as a rubbing tool, and pushing a ball into an enclosed space and then releasing it. These and other categories of play are spontaneously produced by the dolphins and need no reinforcement by trainers with rewards of food or praise.

SOCIAL PLAY

In some species, specific social signals are used to denote that what follows is play rather than serious behaviour. Dogs, for example, signal their readiness to play by dropping down on their forelegs and wagging their tails. In domestic cats, a bout of social play is often initiated by one kitten crouching with its head held low and paddling its back legs before pouncing on another kitten (West, 1974). Chimpanzees have a special 'play-face' – a distinctive facial expression that precedes and accompanies a bout of social play.

Social play is marked by a degree of cooperation between the players. Competition is limited and roles are often reversed. So individuals that are normally dominant in non-playful contexts may allow themselves to adopt a subordinate role during play and vice versa. A mother cat playing with her kitten will sometimes be the object of a playful attack and sometimes initiate it (Mendl, 1988). This exchange of roles during play is particularly striking when members of different species are reared together, such as dogs and cats, cats and rats, dogs and deer, dolphins and whales, and so on.[4] The participants play enthusiastically and frequently exchange roles, as if they share the same set of basic rules for play.

When social play is in full swing, many patterns of 'serious' behaviour are apparent but they are not exactly the same in form or motivation. Playing kittens may pounce on each other, as though fighting or attacking prey, but their biting is soft and when they wrestle their claws are retracted. (This seems to be an inhibition that emerges as the animals get older, because earlier in development they can bite hard and scratch each other.) Similarly, playing monkeys may mount each other, as though sexually, but no actual penetration occurs.

OCCURRENCE IN THE LIFE CYCLE

Despite all the problems with definition, the general consensus is that play is typically something that children and young mammals do. Social play in domestic cats, for example, first occurs at around 3–4 weeks after birth. Meredith West (1974) found that a composite measure of social play rises to a peak 12 weeks after birth and then declines, although some components of social play that involve physical contact peak earlier (Barrett & Bateson, 1978). In wild-living cheetahs, Tim Caro (1995) found that social play involving contact peaks 5 weeks after birth. Other field studies have similarly found play to be largely restricted to periods in early life (e.g. olive baboons: Chalmers, 1980; Southern fur seals: Harcourt, 1991a).

While the occurrence of play tends to decline with the onset of adulthood, it may still be seen in later life. Play is obvious at times in adult domestic cats and dogs. Their behaviour is not just a consequence of domestication, because play in adults has also been seen in many wild species including wolves, coyotes, Cape hunting dogs, gorillas and dolphins (e.g. Kuczaj et al., 2006).[5] And, of course, play is also seen in adult humans, when they have the time and inclination. Adult humans typically play less than children, but we suggest later that they have much to gain from deliberately adopting a more playful approach to life.

SENSITIVITY TO WELL-BEING

Another of the defining features of play that we listed above is its sensitivity to prevailing conditions. In general, play is an indicator of psychological and physical well-being (Held & Spinka, 2011). It is usually the first activity to disappear if an individual is stressed, anxious, hungry or ill. Experimental evidence backs this up. In one study, for example, playing rats that were exposed to cat hair immediately stopped playing or soliciting play, and their play remained suppressed for several days after this mildly stressful experience (Panksepp, 1998). A number of laboratory and field studies have suggested that young mammals that have been short of food play less compared with when they are better fed; examples include squirrel monkeys (Baldwin & Baldwin, 1977) and rock hyrax and tree hyrax (Magin, 1988). Young vervet monkeys in East Africa do not play in dry years when food is scarce, but appear to compensate by playing a great deal when food is plentiful (Lee, 1984). Similarly, gelada baboons play more during rainy periods when food is abundant (Barrett, Dunbar & Dunbar, 1992). In another experimental study, wild-living meerkats were found to play more when they were provisioned with extra food (Sharpe et al., 2002).

Shortage of food tends to suppress play in humans as well. In a comparison of under-nourished and well-nourished children aged 7–18 months in West Bengal, the under-nourished boys (for whom the sample size was adequate, unlike the girls) showed less vigour in their play (Graves, 1976). Similarly, a study of Kenyan toddlers found a correlation between the children's food intake and how much they played (Sigman et al., 1989). Many aspects of poverty, such as a requirement to work, can reduce a child's opportunity for play (Milteer & Ginsburg, 2012). All are a cause for concern, but reduced motivation to play, caused by poor health and poor nutrition, will compound the other problems. As in other species, children's play happens only when basic short-term needs have been satisfied and the individual is free from stress.

INTRINSIC MOTIVATION

The motivation to play has many of the same characteristics as the motivation for other activities such as eating. The more an individual has been deprived of play, the more it will play when given the opportunity, as though compensating for the previous shortfall (e.g. (Jensen, 1999; Wood-Gush, Vestergaard & Petersen, 1990). More saliently, an individual is prepared to work in order to be given the opportunity to engage in play. Opportunities to play are themselves rewarding, reinforcing the activity that provides the individual with the chance to play. In one experiment, for example, an opportunity to play worked effectively as a reward when rats made the correct choice in a maze (Humphreys & Einon, 1981). Like food, the opportunity to play is a natural reinforcer of other behaviour. Moreover, the same neural mechanisms that are involved in food and drug rewards are involved in social play (e.g. Panksepp, 2011).

An individual absorbed in playing seems not to require any external reward. Many experimental psychologists investigating how behaviour is controlled have tended to focus on external rewards or punishments, which are more amenable to experimental manipulation. External rewards such as food are powerful ways of shaping behaviour. In the first half of the twentieth century, B. F. Skinner founded a whole school of research in which animals' responses to different schedules of reinforcement with food were automatically recorded. When the reinforcements occur in a particular context, that context can itself become rewarding. So a food reward delivered after the performance of a particular act may be given only when the trainer has, for example, triggered a device that emits a clicking sound. After a while, the sound alone can be used to reward another act. In the language of experimental analysis of behaviour, the sound is a secondary reinforcer, whereas the food is the primary reinforcer.

Both primary and secondary reinforcers are external and, in the case described, depend on the trained individual being intrinsically motivated to take food. The motivation for learning the rewarded behaviour is said to be extrinsic. In the case of play, particularly when the individual is playing on its own, the motivation is intrinsic – that is, no external reward is needed. In social play the reactions of the play partner may provide an additional reward, increasing the likelihood that the initiator will continue playing. If the partner does not respond playfully, the initiator will stop. Nevertheless, the initiator's behaviour starts spontaneously and may be marked by a characteristic play signal. The spontaneous character of the behaviour is obvious and highlights the distinction between extrinsic and intrinsic motivation.

The various forms of play within a species, and the different ways in which these change with age, suggest that different forms of play are controlled differently (Barrett & Bateson, 1978; Bateson, 1981; Chalmers, 1980; Harcourt, 1991a). Moreover, as play merges with adult behaviour, the motivational systems probably change with age. Aggressive acts can become incorporated into social play, and prey-catching in carnivores can become incorporated into object play.[6]

INDIVIDUAL DIFFERENCES

As in other aspects of their biology and psychology, individuals differ from one another in how much they play and how playful they generally are. Every quantitative study of play finds considerable variation between individuals. This variability might reflect differences in any one of the factors that affect intrinsic motivation, but the characteristic behavioural style of the individual, often referred to as its 'personality', also plays a part. Some individuals tend to be high-spirited even in difficult circumstances, whereas others are typically dour and difficult to rouse into play at any time. Such differences have been found, for example, in chimpanzees (Hoof, 1973) and vervet monkeys (McGuire, Raleigh & Pollack, 1994).

Genes can also affect playfulness. In a comparison of two genetically different strains of rats, one strain (Lewis) consistently played more than the other (Fischer) strain (Siviy et al., 2003). The differences were present even after social isolation. When the Fischer rat pups were fostered by Lewis mothers, they remained less playful than the Lewis pups, suggesting that the behavioural difference in playfulness was due to genetic differences rather than the mother's behaviour.

Behavioural differences between breeds of domestic cats and dogs have been widely described (Hart & Miller, 1985; Mendl & Harcourt, 1988). These differences include differences in playfulness. A large study of domestic dogs found that individuals differed markedly in their playfulness (Svartberg & Forkman, 2002). Behavioural data from over 15,000 dogs of 164 different breeds were used to investigate the existence of personality traits in these animals. Each dog's interest in playing with a stranger was carefully tested. In one test, for instance, the stranger gave the handler a strong piece of rag. The handler dragged the rag on the ground in front of the dog. Before the dog grabbed it, if the dog was willing to do so, the rag was tossed several times between handler and stranger and then thrown away from the dog, which was free to run after and catch it. The dog's reaction varied from no interest in the tossing of the rag to actively playing and following the thrown rag. Statistical analysis of the data for many categories of behaviour revealed the existence of five traits, among which was 'playfulness', meaning in this case propensity to play. Within any one species, many of the behavioural differences between individuals can be attributed to genetic differences (Spady & Ostrander, 2008), but genetic studies that attempt to identify particular genes affecting play behaviour have yet to be carried out.

Differences arising from differences in genes do not, of course, exclude the possibility of large environmental effects. An experiment involving young pigs showed how their experience before the age of weaning could affect the amount that they played more than a month after weaning (Dudink et al., 2006). Starting at around 2 weeks after birth, piglets were exposed to a sound cue that immediately preceded access to an enriched environment containing straw and mixed seeds. These piglets subsequently played significantly more than those in a control group in which the environmental enrichment procedure was not preceded by the sound cue. The results suggested that being able to predict a positive change in their environment reduced the stress of the piglets and, as a consequence, they became more playful.

Males and females in many species show consistent differences in their play, often reflecting sex differences in their non-playful adult behaviour (Meaney & Stewart, 1985). The stick-carrying by chimpanzees that we described earlier, which looks similar to pretend play in children, occurs much more frequently in females than in males (Kahlenberg & Wrangham, 2010). This sex difference could not be explained by a general propensity for females to play with objects more than males, because other types of objects are played with more by males. Males in many species, including humans, also engage in more rough-and-tumble play than do females (Auger & Olesen, 2009; Meaney & Stewart, 1985; Power, 2000). Many behavioural differences between individuals, including differences in play, may be attributed to their sex.

RESPONSES TO ENVIRONMENTAL CONDITIONS

Individual differences in behaviour sometimes represent conditional tactics available to all members of a species. In one set of environmental conditions a form of behaviour appropriate to those conditions is expressed, while in other conditions the individual expresses a distinctly different form of behaviour appropriate to those different conditions (Bateson, Martin & Young, 1981; Caro & Bateson, 1986). The different forms of behaviour are characteristic for the species and their development appears to be triggered by the conditions rather than being learned.

One example of this phenomenon relates to the age at which a young mammal becomes nutritionally independent from its mother and the impact this has on the expression of play behaviour. A considerable body of experimental evidence suggests that early-weaned domestic cats and rats play more with objects than later-weaned animals (Bateson et al., 1981; Bateson, Mendl & Feaver, 1990; Bateson & Young, 1981; Smith, 1991). The evidence suggests that the time of weaning provides the developing young with important information about the nature of the environment in which they will have to live, and thereby triggers a change in their play behaviour. We stress that these results do not contradict the general finding that chronic starvation suppresses play (Bateson, 2000a): the early-weaned kittens and rats in these studies were neither stressed nor deprived of food. Intervening in the mother–offspring relationship to promote early weaning is not equivalent to the whole family experiencing a shortage of food, and the young cats and rats had unlimited access to food after they were weaned.

In the domestic cat, mothers will generally wean their young earlier if their energy loss during lactation is heavy because they have a large litter. Kittens in larger litters show a sharper decline in the rate at which they put on weight at an earlier age than those in smaller litters, indicating earlier weaning onto solid food when the load on the mother is greater (Deag, Lawrence & Manning, 1987). Rats mated immediately after the birth of one litter give birth to pups in the next litter that play more. These pups also start to take solid food at an earlier age (Gomendio et al., 1995). The pups behave as though they anticipate the nutritional burden that will be placed on the mother when she nurses the next litter. A substantial body of research indicates that in mammals the mother's state triggers the long-term expression of a whole suite of characteristics in her offspring (Bateson & Gluckman, 2011). The relevance of the early weaning studies is that individual differences in the amount of play may reflect tactical responses to local conditions, by which the developing individual gathers valuable experience through playing while it still has the opportunity to do so. The functional significance of this variation in play is considered further in the next chapter.

NEURAL CORRELATES OF PLAY

In their book *The Playful Brain*, Pellis and Pellis (2009) suggest that play represents 'the last great challenge to the neural sciences'. We suspect that this claim is a trifle exaggerated, since other major challenges to the neurosciences include chronic pain, depression, addiction, anxiety, Alzheimer's and schizophrenia. Obviously, neural activity in the brain is necessary for play to occur, although the detailed mechanisms by which the brain controls play remain largely unknown. Various neurotransmitter systems, including opioids, endocannabinoids, dopamine and noradrenaline, are known to have an important modulatory role in the production of play behaviour – as they do in most other forms of behaviour (Trezza, Baarendse & Vanderschuren, 2010). In general, the problems of relating particular brain states to particular forms of behaviour are not trivial. How does one distinguish between different explanations? Even the use of brain scanning to determine which parts of the brain are most active when an individual behaves in a particular way is fraught with difficulties. The parts that 'light up' may not be the brain regions that actually control the behaviour. Techniques have been developed to overcome these methodological difficulties, using different approaches to eliminate different subsets of possible explanations (Bateson & Martin, 1999). This approach, which has not yet been used in neurological studies of play, is equivalent to triangulation.

Research has, however, provided some clues about which parts of the brain may be most directly involved in the expression of play behaviour. Experiments on rats, in which small regions of the brain are selectively removed, have shown that the medial prefrontal cortex is necessary for play to occur (Bell et al., 2009). However, the specificity of the effect is not clear. As in many such studies, the lesion may well have a more general effect on behaviour, reducing the expression of various activities besides play. Another experiment, however, suggested a greater degree of specificity (Bell, Pellis & Kolb, 2010). Female rats were kept from the time they were weaned until puberty under one of two conditions. In the control condition, each rat was caged with three juvenile females. In the experimental condition, each rat was caged with three adult females. Young rats housed with adults do not play, even though they experience other normal social situations similar to those of rats reared with rats of the same age. Microscopic examination revealed that in the brains of the rats that had played, the neurons in the medial prefrontal cortex had shorter dendrites. This neurological difference was not found in the orbitofrontal cortex, which did, however, display an effect of the number of same-aged peers present. Although both parts of the cortex showed plastic changes, the effect of play was specific to just one of them – the medial prefrontal cortex. This region was less well developed in the play-deprived rats and had more connections than in animals that had played.

The presence of *more* neural connections in the play-deprived rats may seem counterintuitive, but it does make sense when considering how the brain develops. A notable feature of the mammalian nervous system is the superabundance of connections between neurons at the beginning of development. As the individual develops, many of these connections are lost and many cells die (Bus, Sun & Oppenheim, 2006). Those neural connections that remain active are retained and the unused ones are lost. This sculpting of the nervous system by experience reflects the steadily improving efficiency of the body's perceptual, command and control systems. The play deprivation in the study by Bell et al. (2010) appeared to interfere with this experience-dependent removal of neural connections in the brain, although it remains possible that the presence of adults might have affected neuronal connections in some other unknown way. Proving that particular brain structures are both necessary for, and specific to, a particular form of behaviour is seldom easy.

In Chapter 10 we describe the effects of various psycho-active drugs on playfulness and creativity. Since the sites of action in the brain of these drugs are often reasonably well known, this type of research can provide some insight into the neural basis of the behaviour.

CONCLUSIONS

Having noted the longstanding difficulties in defining play, we propose a definition based on five core features: intrinsic motivation, protected context, novel combinations, repetition, and sensitivity to conditions. These diagnostic criteria define play in the sense that most biologists and psychologists would recognise it, as distinct from the very broad, colloquial usages of 'play'. We further distinguished between play and playful play through the addition of a sixth feature – the presence of a particular positive mood.

Many different forms of play behaviour are observed. In animals, play with objects and play with other individuals peak at different stages of development, with social play appearing before object play. While play is mainly associated with the juvenile period of life, adults also play. Sex differences in the form and frequency of play are often observed and individuals of the same sex within a species may differ greatly in how much they play. Some of these differences are due to genetic differences and some are due to differences in individuals' experience, particularly when environmental conditions trigger a distinctive trajectory of development. Research on the neural basis of play is still in its infancy but studies have implicated the medial prefrontal cortex as being especially important.

3

The functions of play

In this chapter, we consider the general question of play's biological function or functions – in other words, what play is *for*. This question is not directed at the individual's immediate motivation; it is concerned with how various aspects of play increase the individual's chances of surviving and reproducing. The biological costs of play, such as they are, must presumably be outweighed by its biological benefits, otherwise animals that played would be at a disadvantage compared with those that did not, and play would not have evolved. Our central concern in this book is the link between play and creativity and hence innovation. Inasmuch as this link brings benefits in terms of enhancing the organism's chances of survival and reproduction, the way in which play does this is one of its biological functions. However, many other functions have been proposed for play besides enhancing creativity.

THE FOUR WHYS

For most behavioural biologists, the difference between motivation and function is obvious, but some psychologists are uninterested in or unaware of the distinction made by Niko Tinbergen (1963). He recognised that biologists working on behaviour focus on different types of problem. Some want to know, for instance, how the expression of a particular character is controlled, while others want to know how it benefits the organism. Tinbergen pointed out that four fundamentally different types of problem are raised in biology: mechanism, development, function and evolution. These can be expressed in terms of four questions about any feature of an organism:

- How does it work?
- How did it develop during the lifetime of the individual?
- What is it for?
- How did it evolve over the history of the species?

In the case of a fully formed feature of an organism, including forms of behaviour, the mechanism and function are current, while evolution and individual development are historical (Martin & Bateson, 2007). In this chapter we look at the functions or utilities of play, and in the next chapter we consider how the various components of play might have evolved and how they might, in turn, affect subsequent evolution (see also Martin, 1984a).[7]

MANY HYPOTHESES

In the history of thinking about the biological functions of play, a very large number of different hypotheses have been offered (e.g. Baldwin & Baldwin, 1977). When young animals playfully practise the complex movements they will use in earnest later in life, their play is often thought to improve the coordination and effectiveness of these adult behaviour patterns. The potential benefits may be more short term, however. The dashes and jumps of a young gazelle when it is playing bring benefits that may be almost immediate, as it faces the threat of predation from cheetah or other carnivores intent on a quick meal, and needs considerable skill when escaping (Gomendio, 1988). The cheetah's own young also need to acquire running and jumping skills early in life in order to evade capture by lions and hyenas (Caro, 1995). Even though the benefits of play may be immediate in such cases, they may also persist and enhance the crucial survival skills needed in adult life.

Many other benefits have been proposed over the past century and longer. Play, it is said, may enhance an individual's physical coordination, its ability to recognise kin, or its ability to cooperate with others and co-exist with other members of its own species. Play may allow the young animal to simulate, in a relatively safe context, potentially dangerous situations that will arise in its adult life. (In Chapter 10 we consider how a similar function has been proposed for dreaming.) The young animal may learn from its mistakes, but does so in relative safety. According to this view, play exerts its most important developmental effects on risky adult behaviour such as fighting, mating in the face of serious competition, catching dangerous prey, and avoiding becoming someone else's prey. In line with this idea, behaviour that resembles fighting and prey-catching is especially obvious in the play of cats and other predators, whereas intrinsically safe activities such as grooming, defecating and urinating have no playful counterparts. Play, it has been suggested, may increase the individual's knowledge of its home range. It may make an individual more resistant to stress, or enlarge its behavioural repertoire, making it more flexible and better able to adjust to new conditions. Or, as we suggest here, play can help to generate creative solutions to challenges. We examine the main hypotheses about the functions of play in a little more detail before considering how they might be tested.

Most theories about the functions of play have focused on its role in enabling the developing individual to acquire and practise complex physical skills and, by so doing, fine-tune neuromuscular systems. Other theories, reflecting how young animals play with each other, have emphasised how the individual develops social skills and cements its social relationships in the course of play, or improves its capacity to compete and cooperate with other members of its own species (Bekoff, 1976; Geist, 1978).

Given the energetic character of play in animals, many writers have supposed that it provides physical exercise that facilitates the development of adult musculature. This was the view of Groos (1898), who was one of the first to write about the subject. Brownlee (1954), who studied cattle, suggested that play exercises the muscles used in escape, fighting and reproduction later in life, while Robert Fagen (1981) proposed, among other things, that the activities involved in energetic play would also train the young animal to improve its physical balance.

Active engagement with the environment is likely to bring other less obvious benefits, because objects are literally examined from different viewpoints while playing – and objects in the real world rarely look the same from different angles (Bateson, 2000b). Once experienced, such objects are more easily recognised whichever way they are seen. Playing with them is likely to help the individual to construct a working knowledge of the environment: identifying objects, understanding causal relationships, and discovering that things are found when stones are turned over and the world is rearranged. Yet another hypothesis is that young animals benefit from familiarising themselves with the topography of their local terrain as a result of playing in it (Stamps, 1995). Simply knowing the locations of important physical features will usually help, although it will not guarantee safe passage around obstacles when escaping from predators or chasing prey. The seemingly playful movements ensure that, when things become serious, the animal will be better able to negotiate, efficiently and automatically, the obstacles that clutter its familiar environment. As it does so, it will be able to monitor the positions of predators, prey or potentially hostile members of its own species.

Play has features that make it suitable for finding the best way forward in a world of conflicting demands. In acquiring cognitive skills, individuals are in danger of finding suboptimal solutions to the many problems that confront them. In deliberately moving away from what might look like the metaphorical final resting point, each individual may end up somewhere better. Play may therefore fulfil a probing role that enables the individual to escape from false endpoints, or local optima (Bateson, 2011). An analogy is a mountain surrounded by lesser peaks. A climber might get to the top of a lesser peak only to discover that they must descend again before scaling a higher one. When stuck on a metaphorical lower peak, it can be beneficial to have active mechanisms for getting off it and onto a higher one. In practice this means that play is an evolved mechanism for uncovering possibilities that are better than those obtained without playing. We discuss in Chapter 10 how the random thought associations that occur in dreaming, or in altered states of consciousness invoked by some psychoactive drugs, may serve a similar end of generating new, and occasionally better, outcomes.

Yet another function of play may be to prepare for the unexpected. A kitten playing with a ball pats it between chair legs, under sofas and so forth, seemingly making the job of controlling the ball more difficult for itself – an aspect of play known as self-handicapping. Spinka, Newberry and Bekoff (2001) speculated that this type of experience, in which the player deliberately creates obstacles and surprises for itself, provides training for awkward and unexpected situations in adulthood. They also suggest that play might enhance the ability of animals to cope emotionally with the unexpected. When animals play they might rehearse behavioural sequences in which they lose full control over their locomotion and need to recover quickly. Playing provides them with experience of rarely occurring movements, such as might happen when an animal is fleeing from a predator and must regain forward motion after swerving awkwardly.

Self-handicapping during social play involves a bigger, stronger individual restraining itself when playing with a smaller, weaker playmate. The self-handicapping is not always completely symmetrical. In a study of adolescent and adult dogs, higher-ranking and older dogs generally showed a higher proportion of attacks and pursuits, and a lower proportion of self-handicapping, than lower-ranking and younger play partners (Bauer & Smuts, 2007). This may be a case where play becomes serious and the stronger dog exerts its authority.

Theories about play leading to the acquisition of knowledge and resilience, with long-term benefits, are distinct from the idea of play as a mechanism for generating novel and creative solutions, which is the primary thrust of this book. The suggestion that versatility, flexibility and creativity in adulthood are causally linked to play earlier in life has a long history going back at least as far as Herbert Spencer (1872). Fedigan (1972) suggested that the animal puts out 'as many tests or probes of the environment as possible, to innovate'. Similarly,

Fagen (1974) wrote that: 'Playful recombination of motor patterns and responses into new sequences could, like rearrangement of genetic material, tend to increase the phenotypic variability of an animal's offspring.' It is important to distinguish, as these authors have done, between gaining flexibility, becoming more adaptable, and rearranging actions or thoughts to create novel solutions – a potential mechanism behind creativity and innovation. Flexibility and versatility are about being able to deploy a variety of different responses, and adaptability is about being able to deploy an appropriate response to a challenge, whereas creativity is about generating novel behaviour that might provide a new solution.

Many theories suggest, then, that the experience, skills, problem-solving abilities and knowledge needed for serious purposes later in life are actively acquired or enhanced through playful engagement with the environment, including other members of the species. In this sense, some forms of play may be regarded as a metaphorical developmental scaffolding used to construct adult behaviour (Bateson, 1981). Like the scaffolding used to erect a building, play behaviour disappears from the adult repertoire once the job of assembling the components of adult behaviour is complete. The scaffolding analogy is clearly imperfect, since many adults continue to play, albeit at lower rates than young animals, although – as any athlete or musician knows – continued practice is essential to maintain their skills. Moreover, the scaffolding analogy does not adequately describe some of the other proposed functions of play, particularly its impact on creativity. If play has many different potential functions, as we believe it does, then the plethora of explanations is hardly surprising.

TESTING HYPOTHESES ABOUT FUNCTION

Distinguishing between the many different hypotheses about the biological functions of play is difficult because the presumed benefits are usually thought to be delayed, appearing later in the individual's lifetime. The utility to an individual of a characteristic that enhances its chances of surviving and reproducing is testable in principle, but is seldom tested in practice.

Solid evidence for the biological benefits of play has not been readily forthcoming. Martin and Caro (1985) were critical of the assumption that play must necessarily be highly beneficial. They examined three types of evidence: correlations between play and beneficial outcomes; effects of experimental enhancement or deprivation of play experience; and arguments from optimal design about whether the observed features of play are consistent with its proposed function. At the time they were writing, none of these strands was backed up by convincing evidence that play actually provided tangible benefits or increased the chances of survival or reproductive success. Martin and Caro (1985) suggested two reasons for the paucity of examples (beyond the obvious reason that relatively few studies had then been carried out). One possible reason was that play in fact had no major benefits. Another possible explanation used the systems theory concept of 'equifinality', or reaching the same endpoint by different routes. The idea here is that an individual deprived of play would find other ways of obtaining the beneficial experience. The mechanisms involved in behavioural development do tend to be redundant, so that if an endpoint is not achieved by one route it may be achievable by another (Bateson & Martin, 1999). Playing when young may be one way to acquire knowledge and skills, but not the *only* way. The individual might, for example, delay acquisition of these skills until it is adult. However, when such experience is gathered without play, the process may be more costly and difficult, even if it is not impossible.

Since Martin and Caro wrote their review three decades ago, the picture has changed. First, studies of animals in their natural habitat have found that the biological costs of play can be very considerable, implying that play must have compensatory benefits or it would not have evolved. Second, individuals that play more have in some cases been found to be more likely to survive.

Before considering this more recent empirical evidence, it is worth noting that Martin and Caro's critical analysis caused considerable rethinking about the function of play. Indeed, Brian Sutton-Smith (1997) was impressed by the uncertainty and ambivalence among the principal theorists on animal play and noted the immense empirical as well as theoretical ambiguity that surrounded the study of play. He asked: 'Is it not possible to think of the adaptive function of play as being intrinsic and independent of its usefulness for other more extrinsic forms of survival?' We agree that it is possible to think about the *features* of play as being independent of their utility, but not their *adaptive function*, which can be determined only in terms of survival and reproductive success.

Play has real biological costs for the player. Animals expend more energy and expose themselves to a greater risk of injury and predation when they are playing than when they are resting. Play also makes them more conspicuous and less vigilant. For example, young Southern fur seals are more likely to be killed by sea lions when they are playing in the sea than at other times when they are in the sea (Harcourt, 1991b). Such enhanced risks of predation may explain why golden tamarin parents are more vigilant when their offspring are playing (de Oliveira et al., 2003).

Tim Caro (1995) has documented the risks to wild-living cheetah cubs when they are playing, including the opportunity costs of not doing other things, injury, becoming separated from their mother, and disruption of the mother's hunting. The play behaviour of cubs that had left the den was never observed to result in long-term injury or separation. One of us, when observing cheetahs with Tim Caro in the Serengeti National Park in Tanzania, watched a mother stalking a gazelle. Caro, who was a very experienced cheetah watcher, whispered: 'That gazelle has only two more minutes to live'. At that point the mother's playful cubs rushed up, the gazelle fled and the hunt was ruined. Here, then, was one example of play exerting real costs by interfering with the important business of obtaining food. Caro rarely saw this happen: in 478 failed hunts, he saw only 7 disrupted in this way. But when it did happen, the cost to the cubs of losing a meal could be significant.

If play is beneficial, as the evidence suggests it must be, then it follows that depriving the developing individual of opportunities for play should have harmful effects on the outcome of its development, other things being equal. Other things rarely *are* equal, however, and depriving an animal or child of play may also deprive it of other crucial experiences necessary for normal development. Moreover, the individual may acquire the experience in other ways besides playing. Studying such effects experimentally can therefore lead to inconclusive results, as was found in an early study of play experience in domestic kittens (Caro, 1980). Eleven kittens between 4 and 12 weeks old were repeatedly given the opportunity to play with toys. The kittens were given a total of 34 exposures to the toys, each lasting 30–40 minutes. These kittens were reared with their mothers and littermates and had unlimited opportunities for social play. Eight control kittens were similarly reared with their mothers and littermates but received no opportunities to play with toys. All the kittens were individually tested on their ability to catch and kill four different types of live prey when they were 6 months old. No clear-cut differences were found between the two groups. Caro recognised the difficulty of interpreting negative evidence and accepted that his results might be explained in a variety of ways. The control kittens might have received enough relevant experience playing with their littermates, or they had been able to play with unintended toys in their pens, such as wood-shavings. Or perhaps the experimental group's experience of playing with toys was irrelevant to prey-catching. Or the measures of prey-catching that Caro used, combined with the small sample sizes, might not have been sufficiently sensitive to detect subtle differences in skill that could nonetheless be important in the real world.

Negative evidence continued to accumulate elsewhere. In field studies of wild meerkats, the amount of play by the young did not affect subsequent fighting success in 76 individuals from 14 groups (Sharpe, 2005a), nor enhance social cohesion in 55 individuals from 7 groups (Sharpe, 2005b), nor affect subsequent partnerships formed when meerkats disperse from the natal group (Sharpe, 2005c). As Lynda Sharpe pointed out, her evidence did cast doubt on some of the favourite explanations for play. Perhaps she did not measure the right outcome variables. Or perhaps even those individuals who played less still played enough to secure a long-term benefit and, once a given threshold was exceeded, further play did not add value or affect other aspects of adult behaviour. The difficulty with negative findings is that the absence of evidence is not evidence of absence.

Some studies, however, have found measurable consequences of manipulating animals' play experience. In one such study, play interactions between rats enhanced their subsequent ability to respond to novel situations (Einon & Morgan, 1976). In a later experiment, rats were reared from 20 to 50 days after birth in one of three conditions: in pairs; or in isolation, with or without the opportunity to receive up to an hour of social play each day (Einon & Potegal, 1991). The young rats were rehoused in small groups at 50 days of age, when the frequency of play normally starts to wane, so that they were not socially isolated at the time of testing. They were then tested for how they responded defensively at 80–100 days old when placed into the home cage of another adult. (Adults usually respond aggressively to an intruder.) The play-deprived animals spent significantly more time immobile after they had been attacked than did animals of the two groups that had not been deprived of play experience. The increased immobility associated with play deprivation was not caused by baseline differences in emotionality, such as those elicited by a novel environment or by the presence of a strange animal, or by non-social aversive stimuli. These experiments suggest that the play-deprived rats' immobility was restricted to situations involving pain coupled with close proximity to, and contact with, another rat. Since no other differences in defensive behaviour were observed, the maladaptive effect of play deprivation would seem to be specific. Sergio and Vivien Pellis (2009) suggested that play helps rats to refine the ability to deal with potentially threatening and stressful situations. Even so, the play-deprived rats may have suffered from some other, unintended form of deprivation that led to their subsequent behavioural abnormalities. If being deprived of play in early life does indeed adversely affect the individual's capacity to cope in a competitive world, depriving children of opportunities for play-fighting may have unintended consequences. Through playing in this way, children may learn how to cope with their own and other people's aggression and violence (see Chapter 8).

Another approach to identifying the biological functions of play relies on uncovering correlations between the behaviour of young animals and their subsequent survival and reproductive success in the natural environment. In one such study, Fagen and Fagen (2004) tracked the play behaviour and longer-term survival of the offspring of 11 families of individually identified, free-ranging brown bears in Alaska. The results showed that cubs who had played more during their first summer survived better from the first summer to the end of their second summer. This apparent link between play and survival could have arisen for a variety of reasons, so the Fagens analysed potential confounding factors: the cubs' condition, pre-natal and first-year availability of salmon (an important food resource for bears), and maternal characteristics. Controlling statistically for these factors, they confirmed that the more the bears had played when they were cubs, the more likely they were to survive to their first year.

In a subsequent study, Fagen and Fagen (2009) found that this association between the amount of play and subsequent survival persisted into later years of the bears' lives when they reached independence. The amount of play accounted for 35% of the variance in survival. Just how play benefited the bear cubs could not be determined from the data. However, the Fagens suggested that much pre-adult mortality might result from events occurring during the stressful environmental conditions of winter hibernation and early spring. Resistance to cold exposure and infectious disease might be involved. It is possible that play helps to produce an individual that is more resilient, both behaviourally and immunologically. If so, the individual would be better able to withstand stress in ways that its observable physical condition alone would not predict. In other populations or species, these same factors could still be important but in different ways; for example, in mediating the development and performance of behaviour patterns involving predator avoidance and defence, which necessarily involve cognition and emotion.

Further evidence that play can improve an individual's subsequent chances of survival came from a study of feral horses (Cameron et al., 2008). The important finding of this study was that those individuals who played more when young survived better and had better body condition as yearlings. In both studies of free-living bears and horses, it remains possible that some unknown third variable might have produced the observed links between play and survival. The individuals that played less may have been less healthy from the outset in ways that were not observable. Nevertheless, the results do lend support to the view that playing when young produces benefits later in life.

ALTERNATIVE TACTICS

While the energy costs of play may not be great (Martin, 1984b), an animal that is short of food makes energy savings when it can do so and gives relatively low priority to play (Martin & Caro, 1985). We noted in Chapter 2 that play is especially susceptible to poor health or poor nutrition – indeed, its sensitivity to prevailing conditions is one of its defining features. Animals and children generally do not play when they are ill, hungry or stressed. How, then, can the increased object play of early-weaned cats and rats, described in Chapter 2, be explained in terms of increasing the animal's chances of surviving and reproducing?

If cues from the mother indicate that the family will break up earlier, because the mother cannot sustain her investment in caring for her offspring, the young animal would benefit by boosting its play experience while it is still able to do so in a safe environment (Bateson & Young, 1981). Enforced independence at an earlier age would mean the young animal would have to start hunting for its own food at an age when it could otherwise have been honing its predatory skills by playing. To mitigate these ill-effects of curtailing play, the early-weaned young might play more while they still had the opportunity to do so, compared with offspring that were on track to be weaned later. Such a conditional response, if it happens, would imply that those individuals who played more in response to being weaned earlier were more likely to survive than those that did not.

In an attempt to test this hypothesis, the development of predatory behaviour was studied in kittens that had experienced early, normal or late weaning (Tan & Counsilman, 1985). Early weaning was simulated by gradual separation from the mother starting at 4 weeks after birth, while late-weaned kittens were left with their mothers and were denied access to solid food until the ninth week. The results showed that early-weaned kittens developed predatory behaviour sooner than normally and late-weaned kittens and were more likely to become mouse-killers at an early age, even though they were given plenty of food. The functional significance of such a conditional response needs to be examined under natural conditions to confirm that it is real. Even so, it seems likely that by responding to cues from its mother, an individual is able to move along a developmental route that is appropriate to the conditions it is likely to encounter in later life. Early weaning by the mother may indicate that environmental conditions are poor and the kitten therefore needs to gather experience by playing in a protected environment while it is still able to do so.

More generally, an adaptive response by the offspring to the nutritional state of its mother has been a major feature of the scientific literature on the developmental origins of human health and disease (e.g. Bateson et al., 2004; Gluckman & Hanson, 2006). An individual that responds appropriately to its mother's current condition fares better than one that does not, so long as environmental conditions do not change. If, however, its characteristics no longer match the environment it eventually encounters, then its chances of survival are likely to be reduced. Usually the individual benefits by adjusting the trajectory of its development so that its phenotype is best matched to the anticipated environment. The alternative pathways that lead to different developmental patterns of play in cats, depending on when they were weaned, may be one example of a more general phenomenon.

CONCLUSIONS

Attempts to demonstrate that any one of the many plausible explanations for the functions of play is correct have proved extraordinarily difficult, despite much thought and effort. Nevertheless, recent evidence does suggest that animals that play more when young are more likely to survive in the natural environment. Given the wide variety of forms of play, it may well be that many or most of the postulated benefits of play are real.

Our aim is to examine how play and playfulness may enhance creativity and innovation in humans. The survival and reproductive success of individuals may not be the most pressing issues in the daily lives of affluent people in technologically advanced societies. But creativity and innovation clearly do matter, both now and in the past. The creative ability to find novel solutions could have made a big difference to the ancestors of present-day humans in terms of surviving and reproducing. In the present context, the survival of business organisations that depend on innovation for their success could be affected by how much they encourage playfulness, and hence creativity, in their employees. This is a topic to which we return in Chapter 7.

4
_____

Evolution and play

This final chapter on biological aspects of play forms a further backdrop to our investigation into the links between play, playfulness, creativity and innovation. No serious biologist disputes that organisms have changed over geological time or that they continue to change, such as when insects acquire resistance to pesticides or bacteria acquire resistance to antibiotics. Other organisms have become extinct, many of them in the last decade. What requires explanation is the way in which these evolutionary changes take place. Darwin observed that since members of a species differ from each other, some are more likely to survive and reproduce than others. If the characteristics of these individuals were inherited by their offspring, the descendants would be better adapted to their environment than individuals that did not have those characteristics. So, by the process he termed 'natural selection', lineages would evolve. What then can be said about the evolution of play and playfulness?

SURPLUS ENERGY

In writing about the biology of art, Desmond Morris (1962) suggested that artistic expression became possible when animals had evolved to the point where they had enough surplus energy to engage in it. Gordon Burghardt (2005) developed this idea in relation to play. He suggested that four main factors might have been necessary for the evolution of play.

1. The animals had sufficient metabolic energy to engage in the sustained vigorous activity that typifies play.
2. They were buffered against serious stress and food shortages.
3. They needed to be sufficiently aroused to use the surplus energy in play.
4. The animals were likely to benefit from the experience obtained through play.

As noted earlier, birds and mammals provide the most striking examples of play. What is special about these animals compared with, say, fish or reptiles? Mammals and birds are warm-blooded, and parental care of the young is generally extended. A necessary condition for the evolution of play might therefore have been a protected period in the life cycle when an individual could safely engage in such activity – which comes back to a core feature of play, namely that it occurs in a protected context. The longer the period of pre-adult development, the greater the opportunity to benefit from play and the more complex the resulting behaviour. That at least is the hypothesis. We shall consider how such ideas might be tested.

ONE BENEFIT LEADING TO OTHERS

Once they had evolved, various aspects of play could have conferred different benefits. As outlined in the previous chapter, some aspects of play in some species are probably concerned with honing the nervous system and musculature, some with developing social skills, some with perfecting predatory skills, and so on. From our standpoint, however, the most interesting proposal is that play may have opened up new possibilities – in other words, that it was a source of creativity beneficial to the individual by enabling it to discover new ways of dealing with an ever-changing environment. If this is correct, then older animals should be better able to solve problems set by the environment (or by scientists). Some evidence in line with this prediction came from a study in which novel foraging tasks were presented to family groups of callitrichid monkeys in zoos. Older monkeys were significantly more likely than younger monkeys to be the first to solve the tasks (Kendall, Coe &

Laland, 2005). For animals living in social groups, an additional advantage could have been that some individuals could acquire skills or new ways of doing things by copying other individuals who had already discovered them through play.

Discovering a new form of behaviour through play is a type of creativity. Another type of creativity is applying existing forms of behaviour in new ways. The natural world provides potential examples. When describing the novel capacity of certain birds to open the foil tops of milk bottles left outside houses, Hinde and Fisher (1951) suggested that the birds deployed motor patterns that were normally used in other circumstances; in this case to search for food by tearing at the bark of trees. Hinde and Fisher argued that tearing at bark was a motor pattern that had evolved through Darwinian selection and, when used to tear open the tops of milk bottles, did not require invention by the pioneering individuals. This would explain why other birds were able to copy the bottle-opening pioneers so quickly. However, redeploying the existing motor pattern from trees to bottle tops was itself creative and became a successful innovation, resembling what we suggest may happen through certain forms of play.

More generally, play was clearly not the *only* way for young animals to learn to recognise members of their social group, acquire knowledge of local culture, or become accustomed to their local environment. Animals are patently able to acquire these and other forms of experience without playing. Nevertheless, such outcomes might still have been beneficial consequences of play after it had evolved. They may not have been central to the evolution of play but, once it had evolved, the additional benefits were a bonus. The young animal was able, with no extra cost, to acquire information or hone skills in the course of playing for other reasons, such as practising skills needed in adult life. Gordon Burghardt (2005) postulated a process by which simpler forms of play with restricted benefits could lead, in the course of evolution, to more complex play with more extended benefits. The precursors of play might have been spin-offs from other activities and were then co-opted for one of the proposed benefits of play. As evolution proceeded, and play became more complicated, the benefits may have multiplied. On this argument, most or all of the suggested current benefits of play might turn out to be real. The experience, skills and knowledge needed for serious purposes later in life may all be acquired actively through playful engagement with the environment, including interactions with other members of the species. An important feature of this scheme for our thesis is that the final stage in the evolutionary process produced cognitive resources for generating novel behaviour and creativity.

Creativity is about breaking away from established patterns. Creative people perceive new relations between thoughts, or things, or forms of expression that would normally seem utterly different. They are able to combine them into new forms, connecting the seemingly unconnected. Play is also about breaking away from established patterns and combining actions or thoughts in new ways. Play is an effective mechanism, therefore, for encouraging creativity and hence facilitating innovation. Playfully rearranging disparate ideas into novel combinations is a powerful means of gaining new insights and opening up possibilities that had not previously been recognised. It involves doing novel things or having novel ideas without regard to whether they may be justified by a specified pay-off. In subsequent chapters we shall explore these aspects in greater detail.

TESTING EVOLUTIONARY THEORIES OF PLAY

How can theories about the evolution of play be tested? Historical explanations are by their very nature difficult to test. Direct observation is impossible in the case of past behaviour, but multiple lines of inference can provide the basis for robust conclusions. For example, inferences drawn from comparisons between different populations of the same species, or between different taxonomic groups, can be compelling.

Modern comparative biology provides the tools for analysing the degree of difference between taxonomic groups, with the aim of revealing their evolutionary relatedness and when the lineages diverged in the past. Such comparisons may also reveal whether or not the phenotypic similarities are due to evolutionary convergence, where a common problem set by the environment has been solved independently in analogous ways by unrelated lineages. In particular, our increasing understanding of molecular architecture and the potential to read molecular history in genomic sequences, and indeed to recover DNA from fossils, allow for an improved understanding of what might have happened in the past. For example, DNA sequencing of large components of the Neanderthal genome suggests that some interbreeding occurred between Neanderthals and the ancestors of modern humans (Green et al., 2010). As a result, some people now contain within their genomes a small Neanderthal component. This example illustrates how deductions may be drawn from current evidence about past behaviour; namely that individuals of these two lineages mated with each other.

Many well-documented instances exist of where similarities in structure, behaviour or genome reflect common evolutionary origins. Examples include the relationship between the gill arches of fish and the vascular anatomy of the thorax and neck of primates; and the relationship between the bony structure of fins in whales and the limbs of other mammals. Conversely, while the cephalopod eye and the vertebrate eye show remarkable similarities in form, their independent evolutionary origin is demonstrated by the different anatomical relationships between neural innervations of the retina and the light-sensitive cells (Fernald, 2000). In vertebrates, the innervations are from the front of the eye, requiring the optic nerve to pass through the retina and thereby creating a blind spot. In cephalopods, however, the optic nerve runs from the back of the retina and no blind spot is created. We can conclude in this case that the two superficially similar structures evolved separately.

Can similar comparative approaches be used to understand the evolution of play? Where an environmental challenge required greater processing capacity by the brain, this organ would be expected to evolve with greater rapidity. On the simplifying assumption that a bigger brain enables greater learning capacity, the rate of evolution of a species should correlate positively with its relative brain size. This hypothesis was given some support by a study suggesting that the taxonomic groups that are evolving most rapidly, such as birds and primates, also have the biggest brain relative to body size (Wyles, Kunkel & Wilson, 1983). The conjecture is that behaviour expressed by animals with large and complex brains facilitated their rapid evolution.

The hypothesis that large brains permit faster evolution is further supported by the observed correlation between brain size and behavioural innovation in birds. In a groundbreaking piece of research, Lefebvre and colleagues (1997) analysed 322 published reports of innovative ways in which birds obtain food. The taxonomic orders of the birds were related to stand-ardised measures of relative brain size and a strong correlation was found between the relative size of the forebrain and the frequency of occurrence of novel feeding methods. In one exam-ple among many, a herring gull caught small rabbits and killed them by dropping them on rocks or into the sea, where the rabbits drowned. In another case, a crow was observed to place palm nuts in the path of cars, which crushed the nuts, enabling the crow to eat their contents. More recent research on birds has shown that the species with the biggest forebrains relative to other parts of the brain are also the most successful in invad-ing new habitats (Sol et al., 2005). The innovative species also tend to live longer.[8]

The use of tools has been frequently observed in birds and mammals. Members of the crow family and parrot family pro-vide striking examples. The forebrains of these birds are large. Relative to their body size, the brain size of parrots is similar to that of chimpanzees. In primates, a clear relationship has been found between the relative size of 'executive' parts of the brain (the neocortex and striatum) and the use of tools (Reader & Laland, 2002). A comparative analysis of 533 instances of inno-vation, 445 observations of social learning, and 607 episodes of tool use showed that social learning, innovation and tool use were positively correlated with species' relative and absolute 'executive' brain volumes. The study controlled carefully for other factors and strongly suggested that the ability to learn from others, invent new forms of behaviour and use tools played pivotal roles in primate brain evolution.

These associations between brain size and innovation are relevant to understanding how play evolved and, in particular, its role in creativity and innovation. If play is found in widely separated taxonomic groups (which it is), then it follows that play has either evolved many times or has its origins early in evolutionary history. In order to distinguish between these possibilities Reader, Hager and Laland (2011) analysed ecologically relevant cognitive measures from reported instances of behavioural innovation, social learning, tool use, extractive foraging and tactical deception in 62 primate species. The measures were highly intercorrelated, suggesting that social, technological and ecological abilities have coevolved in primates. Reader et al. (2011) concluded that high general intelligence has independently evolved at least four times in primates, with convergent evolution in capuchins, baboons, macaques and great apes (of which humans are one example).

If play leads to creativity, and if more creative individuals are more likely to survive and reproduce, then the necessary conditions for evolution are satisfied.[9] The most creative individuals would on average have more offspring. Some suggestive data from humans show that the most creative poets and artists do tend to have more sexual partners (Nettle & Clegg, 2006). Of course, the number of sexual partners does not translate simply into reproductive success in a modern context, but it might have done so before the age of easy contraception.

PLAY AND ECOLOGY

One of the least well-explored avenues of play research is the relationship of play to the ecological conditions in which animals live. Several authors have proposed that generalist species – those living in a variety of habitats and capable of eating many different types of food – are more likely to benefit from play than specialist species occupying limited ecological niches (Burghardt, 2005). The premise is that the costs of play will outweigh the benefits for the specialists. However, this argument presupposes that the specialist species have no need of the other benefits of play, such as its effects on social relations or the ability to evade predators.

Analysis of the relationship between play and other life-history characteristics is hampered by limited data about which species play (Burghardt, 2005). The difficulty is that knowledge of play in a given taxonomic group is often limited.[10] Gordon Burghardt (in press) and his colleagues are developing ways for testing whether the presence of a particular character increases the chance of evolving another character – for example, whether a feature of a species that generates abundant surplus resources leads to an increased incidence of play behaviour. They have carried out preliminary analyses looking at the occurrence of social play in adult primates, including humans. Their analyses suggest that primates that eat leaves rather than fruits are less likely to engage in social play. This is consistent with the expectations of surplus resource theory, as fruit-eating species should have more surplus resources to use in play.[11]

The trade-off between the benefits of play and its biological costs may explain some of the individual variation found in quantitative studies of play. Some individuals may be more creative than others, whereas others (the innovators) may be better able to exploit the creativity of their fellows in the social group. The distinction we have drawn between creativity and innovation is relevant here. The balance between two types of individuals, creatives and innovators, might be evolutionarily stable. We know of no evidence that would support such a hypothesis, but it should be open to theoretical simulation and empirical testing.

IMPACT OF PLAY ON EVOLUTION

Before leaving the topic of evolution, we consider how play might have affected the behaviour of the descendants of the playing individuals and hence the course of evolution. How could this happen? The nineteenth-century architect of evolutionary theory, Charles Darwin, knew nothing of the molecular processes of inheritance. In this respect he was no different from his contemporaries. He was sometimes tempted into supposing that acquired characters could be inherited. In the mid twentieth century, the genetic mode of inheritance was brought together with Darwin's evolutionary theory in what was called at the time the Modern Synthesis. This conceptual framework became the dominant mode of biological thought, emphatically reinforced by the culture of genetic determinism that has accompanied the explosion of genomic knowledge.

Evolutionary theory itself continues to evolve, integrating the views of the Modern Synthesis with the explosion of observation and theory coming from the developmental, ecological and molecular sciences (Pigliucci & Müller, 2010). Other mechanisms of inheritance have been discovered. These include the transmission across generations of symbiotic bacteria (Gilbert, 2005), direct epigenetic effects involving the passing on of activated and silenced genes to offspring, indirect epigenetic effects such as those transmitted through the mother's behaviour, and social learning (Jablonka & Raz, 2009). A different line of research has focused on synthesising theories of development and those of evolution – the evolutionary developmental biology movement or 'evo–devo' (Amundson, 2005). Aspects of development may involve particular mechanisms that have a fundamental role in the growth of the organism. These 'developmental tool-kits', such as repeating the same basic pattern of expression in separate segments of the body, are thought to affect evolvability. With developmental tool-kits such as segmentation, evolutionary change can be greatly accelerated.

Darwinian evolutionary theory conventionally proposes that evolutionary changes involve a slow accretion through the selection of spontaneously expressed phenotypic elements underpinned by random mutation. However, Darwin also believed that when individual animals learned to perform an activity, generation after generation, the behaviour would eventually be expressed without the necessity for individual learning. He did not explain how such a process might work. The first plausible evolutionary explanation was proposed by Douglas Spalding (1873).[12]

Spalding's mechanism comprised a sequence of learned behaviour patterns followed by the differential survival of those individuals that expressed the behaviour more efficiently *without* learning. To give one example, Galapagos woodpecker finches use cactus spines or small sticks to probe into holes for insect larvae. This behaviour could have been learned initially in the species' history through trial and error. But subsequently, in the course of evolution, the behaviour of picking up and probing with small sticks could have been expressed spontaneously, because those individuals that did so expended less time and effort than those that continued to learn the behaviour again in each generation. The birds that came to express the behaviour spontaneously were therefore more likely to survive and reproduce than those relying on individual learning. Spalding's idea was advanced again by James Mark Baldwin (1896), Conwy Lloyd Morgan (1896) and Henry F. Osborn (1896), all publishing in the same year. Seemingly their ideas were proposed independently of Spalding and, indeed, of each other, although they may have unconsciously assimilated what Spalding had written 23 years before. To avoid confusion about terminology and precedence, Bateson (2006) has suggested that the proposed process be referred to by a descriptive term: the adaptability driver.

Lloyd Morgan's (1896) account of the adaptability driver was particularly clear. He suggested that if a group of organisms respond adaptively to a change in environmental conditions, the modification will recur generation after generation under the changed conditions, but the modification will not be genetically inherited. However, any genetic variation in the ease of expression of the modified characteristic is liable to favour those individuals that express it most readily. Consequently, an inherited predisposition to express the modification will tend to evolve. The longer the evolutionary process continues, the more marked will be such a predisposition. The process starts through learning or some other form of plastic modification within individuals, but this paves the way for a longer-term change in the genes. The Galapagos woodpecker finch that pokes small sticks into holes for insect larvae appears to have a strong predisposition to pick up sticks, but learns from others what to do with those sticks (Tebbich, Sterelny & Teschke,

2010). Eventually the spontaneously expressed behaviour of picking up sticks may be accompanied by the spontaneously expressed behaviour of poking those sticks into holes.[13]

In principle, then, behaviour patterns that were initially acquired by learning could be expressed spontaneously, without learning, in subsequent generations. In a computer simulation, Hinton and Nowlan (1987) demonstrated how learning could greatly accelerate rates of evolution. As they put it: without learning, solving difficult problems is like searching for a needle in a haystack. Learning tells the evolving organisms, metaphorically speaking, that they are getting close to the needle, thereby allowing appropriate genetic change to occur. This work led to a considerable growth in computer simulations investigating whether learned behaviour could lead to spontaneous expression of the same behaviour in subsequent generations. The results have been contradictory, with some of the theoretical analyses suggesting that learning could accelerate evolution and some suggesting that it could have the opposite effect. Paenke, Kawecki and Sendhoff (2009) proposed a general framework that explained both effects. Spontaneously expressing a behaviour that had been learned in previous generations could be costly if it meant that the animal lost all of its ability to learn. The great evolutionary biologist George Gaylord Simpson (1953) believed that this cost was a fundamental objection to the proposed role of behaviour in evolution. Some evidence from fruit flies suggests that he might have been right, at least about simpler organisms (Kawecki, 2010). The benefit of expressing a behaviour spontaneously was found to be outweighed by the cost of losing the capacity to learn about other things. However, Simpson's point is much less cogent when applied to large-brained animals like birds and mammals, with multiple parallel pathways involved in learning. In these animals, the loss of capacity to learn in one way has no effect on the capacity to learn in other ways (Bateson, 2004). This means that the spontaneous expression of behaviour learned in the course of play in previous generations need have no effect in the current generation on the acquisition through play of new experiences.

An ability to cope with complex environmental challenges through learning opens up ecological niches previously unavailable to the animal: a point eloquently expressed by Avital and Jablonka (2000). They suggested that animals use their plasticity to stretch their behavioural repertoire, and the new behavioural elements are then assimilated genetically in subsequent generations. The exposure to novel environments would inevitably lead to the subsequent evolution by means of classical Darwinian processes of morphological, physiological and biochemical adaptations to those niches.

Play leads to a form of plasticity, since by playing an individual is able to acquire skills and understanding of its physical and social environment. Those aspects of play that are creative in solving a problem, or breaking out of local optima, are beneficial to the individual. Such improvements in what could be perceived as cognitive ability would not occur readily by genetic recombination or random mutation, since the probability of all the necessary changes occurring simultaneously would be small. For instance, a squirrel might have discovered while playing that swinging on a branch enabled it to reach nuts that were previously inaccessible, but this beneficial change in its behaviour remains a learned modification. Similarly, dolphins playfully blowing bubbles might have learned that a curtain of bubbles can trap fish. The next step could occur in one of two ways. The discovery made through play by one individual could then spread by social learning. Alternatively, the discovery could have been made separately by many individuals through play, all of them benefiting in the same way. Then, as was postulated in the adaptability driver hypothesis, those individuals that were able to express spontaneously the beneficial trait (swinging on branches, blowing bubbles, or whatever) were able to compete more successfully. To summarise, the suggested chain of events in the course of evolution is as follows:

1.   Each element in a sequence of behaviour is learned by individuals.
2.   Later in evolution, one behavioural element is expressed spontaneously without the need for learning.

3.   Subsequently in evolution, other elements are expressed spontaneously.
4.   Eventually the complete sequence of behaviour is expressed spontaneously.
5.   Once the saving of time and energy costs involved in learning has occurred, the animal is able more rapidly to build up an increasingly complex repertoire of behavioural sequences.

In such a way, new forms of behaviour arising creatively from play could come to be incorporated into the behavioural repertoire of a species through genetic modification. This hypothesis could be tested by examining whether the most playful species have evolved the most rapidly. To our knowledge, this has not yet been done.

We turn in the next chapter to how play and playfulness can exert important influences in human affairs, particularly in the processes of creativity and innovation.

CONCLUSIONS

Play is recognised in many species of birds and mammals. Whether such behaviour has a common origin in reptilian ancestors is a matter of dispute. Alternatively, play might have evolved separately and be linked to warm-bloodedness or, more directly, to the extended parental care found in both taxonomic groups. With time and energy to spare, those individuals that were motivated to exercise their bodies by playing during development would have been at an advantage over those that were not. In such a scenario, the playful behaviour would have spread through the population. Once in place, a cascade of biological benefits could have followed and driven further evolutionary change. Greater benefits from probing the environment could have led to improved cognitive abilities underpinned by more elaborately organised brains. In turn, play behaviour and its underlying neural structures could have facilitated further creativity and innovation, so driving the evolutionary loop to greater and greater complexity. Much of this, although testable, remains a matter of conjecture, but it serves to emphasise that most or all of the postulated benefits of play may turn out to be real.

5

Creativity in humans

Creativity can be defined in different ways. We use 'creativity' here in the sense of generating novel actions or ideas, particularly by recombining existing actions, ideas or thoughts in new ways or applying them in new situations. In our view, it is preferable to consider separately, under the heading of 'innovation', the question of whether those new behaviour patterns or ideas are practically useful and widely adopted by others. For our purposes, creativity is simply about generating novelty and it is a precursor to innovation.

Measures of human creativity have been strongly influenced by J. P. Guilford's (1956) distinction between two styles of thought, which he described as diverging and converging. The diverging individual is more open to new ideas and the converging individual is more critical and analytical. The differences between the two cognitive styles are measured by what is called the Alternate Uses Task. When asked what can be done with, say, a brick, the convergent thinker says it is used for building a wall. The divergent thinker suggests many different uses, such as a doorstop, a hammer, breaking windows, repelling an attacker, grinding up to make red paste, and so forth. Scoring highly on psychological measures of divergent thinking is sometimes regarded as though it were synonymous with being highly creative, but it is of course just one measure of one aspect of human creativity.

Another key figure in the study of creativity has been Paul Torrance (1972). He identified three main components of

creativity, which he referred to as fluency, flexibility and originality. Fluency refers to the number of different ideas that are
generated when a person is asked about alternative uses for a
particular object. Flexibility refers to the capacity to switch
between approaches; someone who generates ideas within
one category will be perceived as less flexible than someone
who generates ideas from multiple sources. Biologists often
refer to the behavioural manifestation of flexibility as adaptability. The third component, originality, refers to the novelty
of the ideas generated and the individual's lack of reliance on
routine or habitual thought. It is possible for somebody to be
fluent without being original, by having lots of conventional
ideas, or original without being fluent, by having one really
groundbreaking idea. A fluent person might come up with a
long list of commonplace uses for an object, whereas an original
person would suggest uses that no one had thought of before
(Runco et al., 2011).

Many other systematic measures of human creativity have
been developed, such as the ability to find non-obvious connections between words. The Remote Associates Test, for example,
involves presenting participants with a set of words such
as *lick*, *mine* and *shaker* (Mednick, 1968). The task is to identify
another word that connects these three seemingly unrelated
ones. In this example, the answer is *salt*. The link between words
is associative and does not follow simple rules of logic, concept
formation or problem-solving, and thus requires the respond-
ent to be creative. The personality characteristic of Openness,
which we shall consider further below, specifically itemises
creativity as one of its defining features (Nettle, 2007). Yet
other assessments of creativity rely on subjective judgements
that the individual has generated something novel.

These varied considerations have led some to argue that
a unitary explanation of what lies behind creativity would be
hard to find. Undoubtedly, human creativity is a complex and
multifaceted set of capabilities. As Batey and Furnham (2006)
pointed out, measuring creativity requires a battery of different psychological tests, since each test measures a different
facet of the ability. The relations between each measure then

need to be investigated. But despite the problems of defining and measuring creativity, consensus can usually be achieved about individual humans or ideas that are judged to be highly creative.

LINKS BETWEEN PLAYFULNESS AND CREATIVITY

Play involves breaking rules. Playful play involves having fun while doing so. From play may emerge a new perspective or cognitive tool that might be used at a later date, possibly in combination with other perspectives or tools, to solve a new challenge. In their different ways, both of these consequences of play are creative. The zoologist George Bartholomew (1982) wrote: 'Creativity often appears to be some complex function of play . . . related to the exuberant behavior of young animals. The most profoundly creative humans of course never lose this exuberant creativity.'

Human history is full of examples of highly creative and playful people. Universally admired as an enormously creative composer, Wolfgang Amadeus Mozart was well known – notorious even – for his playfulness. The high-spirited pranks and jokes were reflected in his music. Robert and Michèle Root-Bernstein (2001) noted that his three-voice canon (KV559) consists of a nonsensical Latin text which when sung sounds like bawdy German. We mentioned in an earlier book how playful Pablo Picasso was in his art (Bateson & Martin, 1999). He was once filmed painting onto glass. The onlooker saw the picture emerge, but viewed from the other side of the glass. Picasso started by quickly sketching a goat and then rapidly embellishing it. Other shapes appeared and disappeared; colours were mixed and transformed. By the end of the film the goat had long since gone and it would have been hard to say what the picture was all about. Picasso had been playing – probably showing off – but clearly enjoying himself hugely.

M. C. Escher (1989) wrote about his art in the following way: 'I can't keep from fooling around with our irrefutable certainties. It is, for example, a pleasure knowingly to mix up two- and three-dimensionalities, flat and spatial, and to make fun of gravity.' Famous products of this approach were his impossible staircases, an idea he got from the medical geneticist Lionel Penrose and his mathematician son Roger (Penrose & Penrose, 1958). Escher wrote: 'They often provided me with new ideas and sometimes an interaction between them and myself even develops. How playful they can be, those learned ladies and gentlemen!'

The philosopher Thomas Kuhn (1962) likened scientific research to play. Whether all research can be regarded as play-like is doubtful, as Kuhn recognised, but many examples of playful scientists are well known. The discoverer of the anti-bacterial properties of penicillin, Alexander Fleming, was famous for his playfulness. He was described, disapprovingly, by his boss as treating research like a game and finding it all great fun. When asked what he did, Fleming said 'I play with microbes ... it is very pleasant to break the rules and to be able to find something that nobody had thought of' (Maurois, 1959). One of the founders of molecular biology, Max Delbruck, formulated his principle of 'limited sloppiness'. Be sloppy enough, he urged, so that something unexpected may happen, but not so sloppy that you can't tell what it was (Judson, 1980). Sloppiness is not the same as playfulness, of course, but they do have in common the willingness to generate novel variations for their own sake and then see what happens. Delbruck was playfully breaking the rules of 'serious' science. Fleming and Delbruck each won a Nobel Prize.

Another famously playful scientist and Nobel prizewinner was Richard Feynman. When Feynman was getting bored with physics at an early stage in his career, he wrote: 'Physics disgusts me a little bit now, but I used to enjoy doing physics. Why did I enjoy it? I used to play with it. I used to do whatever I felt like doing – it didn't have to do with whether it was important for the development of nuclear physics, but whether it was interesting and amusing for me to play with' (Feynman, 1985). He decided that he would play with physics again, irrespective of how important it might be. Then, while he was playing, everything flowed effortlessly and he made fundamental contributions to nuclear physics.

Social play is marked by cooperation between the players. Competition is limited and roles may be reversed, so individuals that are dominant in non-playful contexts may allow themselves to adopt a subordinate role during play. Sometimes the playfulness is explicit, as in Jim Watson's famous account of an extremely important scientific discovery in the early 1950s (Watson, 1968). He and Francis Crick had set themselves the task of uncovering the structure of deoxyribonucleic acid (DNA). DNA was already recognised as a molecule that could faithfully replicate itself and carry information that was crucial to the development of an individual and which could be transmitted from one generation to the next. Watson and Crick were working in the Cavendish Laboratory in Cambridge and the eyebrows of their sober and hard-working colleagues were raised when the pair disappeared for convivial lunches in the Eagle pub and long walks around the colleges. Watson's book *The Double Helix* conveys strongly the playful nature of scientific creativity – the way in which scientists play around with ideas, trying out new combinations and discarding them if they do not work. He and Crick seized upon model-building as a way of rapidly testing different theories of the DNA structure – an idea that the Nobel-prizewinning chemist Linus Pauling had previously used in working out the alpha-helical structure of proteins. The key lay in finding out which atoms would fit next to each other. To do this, Crick and Watson used a set of coloured balls somewhat like children's toys. Watson wrote: 'All we had to do was to construct a set of molecular models and begin to play – with luck, the structure would be a helix'. It was indeed a helix and its paired structure provided the means for the molecule to replicate itself.

Another example of the association between playfulness and scientific creativity comes from Andre Geim and Konstantin Novoselov, who won the 2010 Nobel Prize for physics. The prize was awarded for their discovery of the 'wonder material' graphene – a two-dimensional lattice of carbon atoms which is stiffer and stronger than diamond while also being stretchable and impermeable to liquids and gases. Graphene is a better conductor of heat and electricity than copper and it can be made into transistors that are faster than conventional silicon transistors. The approach that Geim and Novoselov took to their science was instructive. They first made graphene by playing with pencil leads and sticky tape. In 2004 they discovered that they could make sheets of graphene from a fleck of graphite by simply peeling it off with a strip of sticky tape. In a later interview, Geim said: 'A playful attitude has always been the hallmark of my research . . . Fun actually plays quite a minor part, but it certainly helps. Without it you would consider your job a burden. But you also have to do things no one else is doing. Unless you happen to be in the right place at the right time, or you have facilities no one else has, the only way is to be more adventurous.' In the same interview, Novoselov said: 'If you try to win the Nobel you won't. The way we were working really was quite playful.'

Similarly, Daniel Kahneman, who received the Nobel Prize for economics in 2002, wrote about his playful interactions with his friend and colleague Amos Tversky, who would have shared the prize if he had not died some years earlier: 'Amos was always very funny and in his presence I became funny as well, so we spent hours of solid work in continuous amusement. The pleasure we found in working together made us exceptionally patient; it is much easier to strive for perfection when you are never bored' (Kahneman, 2011).

THE IMPORTANCE OF MOOD

A clear link between certain types of positive mood and creativity has emerged from many different studies, even if the results have not always been consistent. As Lyubomirsky, King and Diener (2005) concluded, 'pleasant moods promote original thinking'. In contrast, others have reported that positive moods can inhibit creativity and negative moods can facilitate it (e.g. George & Zhou, 2002). Context is important. To shed more light on the relationship between mood and creativity, Davis (2009) carried out a meta-analysis[14] of the results of 62 experimental studies and 10 non-experimental studies. In general, the results showed that positive mood is indeed linked to greater creativity.

However, the relationship takes the form of an inverted U, reminiscent of the relationship between arousal and performance. Hyper-excitable positive mood states, it would seem, are not conducive to creativity, while moderately positive states are optimal. An important distinction should be recognised between generating new ideas, which is fostered by positive mood, and innovative problem-solving, where other motivational factors such as determination and persistence may play a role (Davis, 2009). This distinction helps to explain why negative moods such as anger or competitiveness are found to assist problem-solving in some circumstances.

During some types of play, individuals may experience a psychological state known as flow, in which they become utterly absorbed in the task they are performing and are oblivious of passing time (Csikszentmihalyi, 1996). Flow is most likely to occur when an individual is performing a challenging task that is just within the reach of their ability. Flow is rewarding, though it would not always be described as pleasurable in the conventional sense of the word. Flow can occur in many situations, both at work and in leisure activities, such as playing a game or a musical instrument, cooking, performing a delicate manual task, climbing a mountain, or conducting surgery on a patient. Those who experience flow sometimes describe themselves as being 'in the zone'. Flow helps to make the activities that produce it intrinsically rewarding.

Intrinsic motivation comes from the pleasure derived from the task itself or from the sense of satisfaction in completing it. An intrinsically motivated person works on solving a problem because the challenge of finding a solution is sufficient reward. Extensive evidence from psychological research shows that people tend to work harder and perform better in many situations when driven by intrinsic rather than extrinsic motivation, especially when performing tasks that are optional. Indeed, some types of extrinsic reward can actually reduce performance. A meta-analysis of the results of 128 published studies examined the effects on intrinsic motivation of extrinsic rewards such as money or sweets (Deci, Koestner & Ryan, 1999). Tangible extrinsic rewards significantly undermined intrinsic motivation and the individuals' interest in the task. Positive extrinsic encouragement, of the type 'Excellent, keep up the good work', maintained the motivation of college students but was less effective with children. In general, many experiments have found that extrinsic rewards can interfere with intrinsic motivation. Those who are intrinsically motivated may become less motivated to do what they enjoy, and less persistent, if an external reward such as money is introduced and later withdrawn.

INDIVIDUAL DIFFERENCES

As in other species, some humans are more intrinsically motivated to do certain things and more creative than others. These traits may be seen as part of their personality. The so-called Big Five personality traits that explain much of the observed variation in human personalities are:

- Extraversion (outgoing, enthusiastic vs. aloof, quiet)
- Neuroticism (prone to stress and worry vs. emotionally stable)
- Conscientiousness (organised, self-directed vs. spontaneous, careless)
- Agreeableness (trusting, empathetic vs. uncooperative, misanthropic)
- Openness (creative, imaginative, eccentric vs. practical, analytical, conventional).

Daniel Nettle (2007) suggested that Openness should be called 'openness to experience' and noted that the tendency towards exploration of complex recreational practices is uniquely predicted by Openness. This dimension of personality captures the distinction we draw between creativity and innovation, since innovation tends to be more strongly related to being organised and analytical.

Hans Eysenck (1995) suggested that creative genius is associated with high scores on a scale he called 'psychoticism', which is related to mental disorders such as schizophrenia and sharp mood swings. An individual's vulnerability to schizophrenia is manifest in a set of personality traits that is now known as schizotypy. Many studies have shown that individuals involved in the creative arts, such as poets and artists, tend to score higher on two dimensions of schizotypal traits (Batey & Furnham, 2008; Nettle, 2002; Schuldberg, 2000). The two dimensions are: having unusual experiences such as perceptual and cognitive aberrations, hallucinations and magical thinking; and impulsive non-conformity, such as violent and reckless patterns of behaviour. Nettle (2006) compared the schizotypy profiles of a large sample of poets, artists, mathematicians and psychiatric patients against the general population. Poets and visual artists had more ideas and were more open to new experiences than members of the general population, and were as distinct from the general population in this respect as were the psychiatric patients.[15] Nettle also found different cognitive profiles among the creative people. While the poets and artists were typically divergent thinkers in Guildford's sense, the mathematicians scored lower than the general population in having unusual experiences and were generally convergent thinkers. They were also more likely to be autistic.

Is creativity associated with psychiatric disorders more generally? Using a massive data set of more than a million Swedish patients, Kyaga et al. (2012) investigated whether patients with a wide range of disorders were more strongly represented in creative professions, defined as those with scientific and artistic occupations. Individuals in creative professions were no more likely to suffer from psychiatric disorders than matched controls, with the exception of bipolar disorder, which was more common in the creative professions. Kyaga and his colleagues did find an association between the creative professions and first-degree relatives of people with schizophrenia, bipolar disorder, anorexia nervosa, and for siblings of people with autism. They also investigated authors, defined as 'people known for writing, who more or less professionally engage in writing ... especially in terms of literary writings'. Being an author was specifically associated with an increased likelihood of schizophrenia, bipolar disorder, unipolar depression, anxiety disorders, substance abuse and suicide.

In a meta-analysis of 83 published studies of personality and creativity in scientists and artists, Gregory Feist (1998) found that these creative people were more open to new experiences, less conventional, less conscientious, more self-confident, more self-accepting, more driven, more ambitious, more dominant, more hostile and more impulsive than less creative people. Some of these characteristics, such as drive and ambition, may be more strongly related to innovation than to creativity. The divergent feature of creativity does not appear to be correlated with measures of intelligence, which is typically associated with a convergent personality (Furnham & Bachtiar, 2008).

Individuals who are more distractible – for example, finding it hard to screen out noises or conversations – are also more likely to be creative (Carson, Peterson & Higgins, 2003). Students who had greater difficulty in ignoring unrelated stimuli were found to be seven times more likely to be rated as 'eminent creative achievers' based on their previous accomplishments. The proposed explanation was that people who have difficulty filtering out extraneous stimuli are more likely to piece together seemingly unrelated ideas.

How is creativity affected by genes? Reuter et al. (2006) described what they called the first candidate gene for creativity. Runco et al. (2011) replicated and extended this work, analysing the alleles of five candidate genes. College students whose genes were assayed took a battery of tests of their creative potential. Fluency in producing alternative uses for objects was significantly associated with differences in the alleles of four genes coding for two enzymes, either a membrane protein or a receptor associated with mood and the reward system of the brain.[16] However, originality, which is a different and in some ways better measure of creativity, was not related to any of the genes under investigation. The authors concluded that the genetic basis of creativity remained uncertain. It is worth adding that the notion of genes 'for' a behavioural characteristic is a convenient but misleading way of describing a developmental process that involves many different factors. The correct way to express the empirical data is in terms of differences in genes being associated with differences in behaviour.

THE RECEPTION OF CREATIVE IDEAS AND INNOVATIONS

As we have already argued, it is useful to distinguish between the generation of new ideas or behaviour patterns (creativity) and their successful implementation and adoption by others (innovation). This distinction can sometimes be hard to draw, however, in the realm of the creative arts, where creativity may not result in practical implementation of any kind. The creative act may, however, be regarded as innovative when the outcome, such as a new style of painting, influences the work of others. The reactions to a supposed act of artistic creativity often lack consensus or stability across time. Critics of the arts usually differ among themselves, as do audiences. A work might be an instant success, only to decline in popularity and be treated as a passing fad. What at one moment may have been considered avant-garde or revolutionary may later be forgotten. Another work might take a long time before it becomes popular and then remain so for a long period thereafter. In an article on the creativity of people who composed operas, Simonton (2000) noted that the successful creative individual has to fit the zeitgeist, or spirit of the times. He or she must generate the right product at the right place and at the right time. Originality is not best measured by popularity.

Steven Johnson (2010) investigated the origins of good commercial ideas, analysing many examples in which major acts of inventiveness had occurred. He classified the examples in two ways. The first was according to whether an *Individual* (or small group) was involved, or whether the invention resulted from a *Network* in which many groups worked on the same problem. The other way of classifying the good ideas was whether the people involved had hoped to make money from their invention (described as orientated towards the *Market*) or had declared no wish to make money from it (*Non-market*). Using this simple classification scheme, Johnson obtained a 2 × 2 matrix. In the *Market/Individual* quadrant he placed people like Willis Carrier, who invented the air conditioner and made a colossal fortune from his discovery. In the *Non-Market/Individual* quadrant he placed people like Tim Berners-Lee, who invented the World Wide Web to the enormous benefit of fellow human beings but with no direct financial benefit to himself. In the *Market/Network* quadrant were placed examples like the type-writer, and in the *Non-Market/Network* quadrant were placed examples like radar. In all, Johnson examined 135 cases dating from the year 1800 to the present. He found that two-thirds of the successful inventions were generated by groups of people rather than a single individual and, contrary to the belief that most invention is driven by market forces, two-thirds arose without an explicit motive to make money.

Johnson argued that innovations arising from good ideas are much more likely to take off when the social conditions are right for their reception. In doing this, he alluded to the bio-logical concept of the 'adjacent possible', formulated by Stuart Kauffman (2000). Kauffman pointed out that the necessary con-dition for each evolutionary burst is a particular combination of events that had not arisen at an earlier stage in evolution. At the most elementary level, hydrogen could not form water without the presence of oxygen. During biological evolution, as the first lipids self-assembled, they started a process that would ulti-mately lead to cell membranes, which would in turn form an envelope within which the first nucleotides might form, lead-ing to the self-replicating RNAs and DNA.

In human creativity and innovation, ideas have their right moment in the sciences as well the arts. For instance, the nineteenth-century Hungarian obstetrician Ignaz Semmelweis observed that the incidence of puerperal fever could be drastically cut by the use of hand disinfection in obstetrics clinics. The fever following childbirth was common in mid nineteenth century maternity hospitals and was often fatal. However, Semmelweis's observations conflicted with the established scientific and medi-cal opinions of the time and his ideas were rejected, partly because Semmelweis could offer no mechanism to explain his findings. His views earned widespread acceptance only years after his death, when the role of bacteria in infection was discovered.

Radical scientific proposals, such as that of Alfred Wegener (1912) about continental drift, have sometimes been ridiculed at the outset, only to become part of the consensus years later. Another famous case was that of Barbara McClintock (1950), whose discoveries about the transposition of genes in the genome attracted widespread scepticism. With later advances in technology, her ideas about 'jumping genes' were finally accepted and she was awarded a Nobel Prize in 1983. The formalised procedures of science generally mean that good ideas are eventually vindicated and bad ones are eventually rejected.

The impact and uptake of a new idea may even be affected by the social status or celebrity of the person associated with that idea. Greater credence is often given to the ideas of an admired person than to those of people of lower status. This human tendency to indulge in 'celebrity worship' may actually make good sense in terms of evolutionary biology, if it is seen as a predisposition to pay attention to and emulate the behaviour of the most successful individuals. During the course of evolution, humans probably did benefit, on average, from aping their most successful peers (Martin, 2005).

WINNOWING OF IDEAS

Two years before Charles Darwin's death, the philosopher and psychologist William James suggested that the process of innovation by humans is analogous to Darwin's account of the evolutionary process of natural selection. Innovation starts with a variety of different ideas, some good but mostly bad. This pool of possibilities, James suggested, is subjected to a winnowing process, leaving only a few that are of any interest. Finally, those ideas that survive are transmitted into the future. A similar concept of innovation has appeared in the writings of others, most notably Donald Campbell (1960), one of whose seminal papers on epistemology was entitled 'Blind variation and selective retention in creative thought as in other knowledge processes'. In much the same vein, Dean Swinton and John Sweller suggested that the creative process is like the evolutionary process by which differential survival follows from a mass of possibilities, some good but most bad. This process, which is known as a genetic algorithm, is used by engineers in developing optimal designs. It relies on generating and then testing a wide variety of possibilities and selecting the one that empirically works best.

CONCLUSIONS

Human creativity is a complex set of capabilities that can be measured in a variety of ways, one of which is the divergent ability to generate many possible uses for an object. Creativity may be separated into the distinct dimensions of fluency, flexibility and originality. The most creative individuals often exhibit great playfulness. Some also exhibit less attractive characteristics such as being more driven, more ambitious, more dominant and more hostile than other people. These features of their personality may be important in translating good ideas into practice. We return to the role of play in creativity in Chapter 7 and explore further how creativity leads on to innovation.

6

Animals finding novel solutions

In this chapter we develop the idea that some of the more interesting cognitive abilities of complicated animals derive from playful experiences earlier in their lives. We freely admit that much of what we propose is speculative and the abilities may also arise in other ways. We begin with a well-known story. In one of Aesop's fables, a crow – half-dead with thirst – came upon a pitcher but found only a little water in it. He could not reach far enough down with his beak to get at the water. After many attempts, he took a pebble and dropped it into the pitcher. He went on dropping in pebbles, raising the water level a little at a time, until at last he was able to reach the water.

The fable has become a reality, not with a crow but another member of the crow family, the rook (Bird & Emery, 2009). In the rook's case the prize was a mealworm lying on the surface of the water in a transparent plastic tube. The rook could not reach the mealworm with its beak but, just as in Aesop's fable, when given a pile of pebbles, the bird dropped them into the water one by one until it had raised the water level enough and could reach the mealworm. The experiment was extended using two Eurasian jays, which are also members of the crow family (Cheke, Bird & Clayton, 2011). The birds were given piles of two different types of object that could be dropped into the water. One pile consisted of pebbles and the other was pieces of cork the same size as the pebbles. The jays quickly learnt to discriminate between the pebbles, which raised the water level, and the corks, which floated on top and did nothing to raise the level. They too used the pebbles to obtain the food. In both cases, the birds appeared to understand and then solve a practical problem with speed and insight, rather than relying on laborious trial and error.

Many years earlier, Wolfgang Köhler (1925) described similar examples of apparently immediate and insightful understanding of problems by chimpanzees. He was director of a research station owned by the Prussian Academy of Sciences on the island of Tenerife and continued to devote his time to the study of captive anthropoid apes when he was interned there during the First World War. When he suspended a banana out of reach of the chimpanzees, they quickly piled wooden boxes on top of each other so that they could reach the banana when they climbed on top of the platform they had created for themselves. In another experiment, Köhler gave the chimps sticks that could be slotted together and used to reach bananas placed more than arm's length away outside their cage. The chimps seemed to have a clear idea of what to do in each case. In Köhler's phrase, they were 'unwaveringly purposeful'. No trial and error was required at the time they solved the problems; they seemed to have insight into the tasks that Köhler had set for them. It was as though they had said to themselves: 'Aha, I know what to do'.

SOLVING PROBLEMS

Many other examples of mammals and birds finding clever solutions to novel problems have been described since Köhler's time. At the Gombe Stream Reserve in Tanzania, Jane Goodall and her collaborators recorded many examples of novel and inventive behaviour in wild chimpanzees (e.g. Kummer & Goodall, 1985). In one case, chimps used large fuel cans in the aggressive charging displays by which rivals are intimidated. One male used the cans in almost all his displays, keeping them in front of him when he charged towards his superiors. Within four months of adopting this new behaviour, he had become the alpha male, having thoroughly intimidated all his rivals and, as far as is known, without taking part in a single fight.

Novel behaviour patterns are sometimes used when one animal appears to deceive another. Jane Goodall described the case of one young adolescent male chimpanzee called Figan. When other chimps were present, Figan rarely managed to get hold of the bananas that had been made available to the group (Kummer & Goodall, 1985). On one occasion, however, he was observed to get up and walk purposefully away from the bananas. His mother followed and others, apparently intrigued, followed after her. Ten minutes later, Figan reappeared by himself and enjoyed free access to the bananas. The human observers thought this was a coincidence, until they saw Figan do exactly the same thing again on four other occasions. It seemed as though he had worked out how to get what he wanted through trickery.

This sort of 'tactical deception' behaviour has been investigated by Whiten and Byrne (1988), who defined it as occurring when an individual is able to use an 'honest' act from its normal repertoire in a different context in order to mislead familiar individuals. They described many examples from primates that looked like genuinely novel behaviour. In one case, a juvenile baboon, who was watching an adult eating a much-prized root, gave an alarm call. Its mother rushed over and drove away the other adult, whereupon the juvenile proceeded to eat the root.

Some birds generate novel behaviour in their courtship displays. Males may add extra syllables to the songs they have copied from their fathers (Marler & Slabberkoorn, 2004). Bowerbirds may add novel items to their bowers (Frith & Frith, 2004). The reward for such creativity is not immediate, although it may lead to greater reproductive success in the end (Madden, 2007).

Novel use of tools has frequently been observed in birds and mammals. Among the birds, members of the parrot and crow families provide some of the best examples. The kea, a New Zealand parrot (e.g. Huber, Rechberger & Taborsky, 2001) and the New Caledonian crow (e.g. Hunt, 1996) are especially remarkable. In one study, the two species were compared on their ability to extract items of food from a box that could be accessed in different ways (Auersperg et al., 2011). Food could be extracted from the box by two techniques requiring the use of tools. One technique involved using a stick to knock the food off a pole so that the bird could reach it. The other required the bird to insert a small ball into an opening so that it would roll down a tube and knock the food off the pole. The birds rapidly worked out how to obtain food in these ways. The crows were better at using the stick, whereas the keas were better with the ball. This difference reflected, in part, the ease with which the two species could handle the tools.

Dolphins and related sea mammals are extraordinarily creative in their ability to generate new forms of behaviour. In one experiment, captive rough-toothed dolphins were trained to produce novel behaviour patterns on command, and were reinforced for doing so (Pryor, Haag & O'Reilly, 1969). This procedure produced significant increases in novel behaviour. It also demonstrated that the dolphins could remember behaviour patterns they had already performed and could learn to produce novel behaviour for which they had not previously been rewarded.

We described in Chapter 2 some of the many and varied types of play behaviour observed by Kuczaj et al. (2006) in captive dolphins. In that study, behaviour patterns were considered novel only if they had not previously been produced by one of the dolphins. If a young dolphin produced a behaviour pattern that no other dolphin had been observed performing, such as tossing a ball against the wall of the pool and catching it in its mouth on the rebound, this was considered to be an example of novel behaviour. We regard the generation of new types of behaviour in this way as creative. Although some novel forms of play were variations of existing behaviour, others were quite different from anything seen before. For instance, one young dolphin discovered over the course of an afternoon that it could take a ball, carefully position it under the opening of a floating box, and release the ball so that it became lodged in the box. Another young dolphin learned how to toss a large wooden disc so that it skimmed across the surface of the water. This behaviour initially startled the other young dolphins that had been observing his play, but it soon intrigued them. They regrouped behind the disc-tossing dolphin and watched his subsequent attempts to skim the disc across the surface of the water.

As the dolphins grew older, their play became increasingly elaborate and they produced more and more novel forms of play. These included swimming upside down on the surface of the water while holding a ball between the pectoral fins, jumping in the air and landing on a ball, using the tail fluke to pin a ball against the bottom of the pool, and pushing a ball along the bottom of the pool. One dolphin, who had picked up a feather, stationed herself in front of an underwater stream of water flowing into the pool; she repeatedly released the feather so that it initially floated away from her and was caught in the stream, which brought the feather back to her, and so on. Another dolphin carried a scarf in its mouth while swimming; it released the scarf, catching it on one of its pectoral fins, then let it go again and caught it with its tail fluke. Altogether, 317 distinct types of novel behaviour had been observed by the time the dolphins were older, many of which were copied by other individuals (Kuczaj et al., 2006).

One particularly interesting technique used by dolphins when playing is to blow bubbles from their blowhole when underwater. Some dolphins become expert at blowing rings of bubbles, with which they then play (Marten et al., 1996). Kuczaj et al. (2006) observed one dolphin using its fluke to hit bubbles that had just been released, swimming under a bubble ring that had just been produced and releasing more bubbles that passed through the ring.

In the wild, dolphins blow a screen of bubbles underwater to drive fish to the surface, where they can catch them more easily (Fertl & Wilson, 1997). Another example of an acquired form of foraging behaviour by dolphins is the use of basket sponges. In Shark Bay, Western Australia, some bottlenose dolphins wear a basket sponge on their beak while lightly scouring the seafloor for prey (Mann et al., 2012; Smolker et al., 1997). The sponge is thought to protect the dolphin's delicate beak. The practice of using sponges in this way is passed down from mother to daughter in a few specific families, which implies that the creative individual who first invented this technique lived some time in the past.

A remarkable instance of novel and unusual behaviour is the cooperative foraging observed in certain small groups of humpback whales in southeast Alaska and the west coast of South America. Many species of marine mammals use bubbles to help them catch prey, but some humpback whales have developed an elaborate technique in which they use a cylindrical curtain of bubbles to surround shoals of herrings. One whale blows a wide circle of bubbles that rises to make a curtain. Other whales emit loud calls that drive the herring towards the bubble wall. As the fish come close to the bubbles, the bubble-blowing whale encloses the wall of bubbles around them, creating a cylinder with the fish trapped inside. The other whales position themselves at the bottom of the cylinder and the herring flee upwards, driven by the whales' calls from beneath them. The whales move upwards together and, as they approach the surface, each one opens its mouth wide and consumes large numbers of fish in a gulp[17] (Wiley et al., 2011). This remarkable and effective feeding technique is seen only in a few specific populations of humpback whales, most notably those feeding in southern Alaska, suggesting that, at one point, it was a creative discovery.

DEVELOPMENT OF NOVEL SOLUTIONS

These and other examples of individual animals producing novel solutions to problems are suggestive of some remarkable cognitive abilities. But how did these abilities develop within those individuals? One possibility is that the behaviour is expressed spontaneously, with little or no dependence on relevant previous experience. In Chapter 4 we discussed how complicated sequences of behaviour could be learned initially but then, in the course of evolution, they come to be expressed without dependence on learning. Such explanations do not, however, readily explain how individual dolphins and whales invent new forms of behaviour, which are then copied by other members of their social group.

Some aspects of the use of tools by New Caledonian crows do seem to be inherited (Kenward et al., 2006). The same is also true for the Galapagos woodpecker finch, which uses cactus spines to prise insect larvae out of holes and has a predisposition to pick up sticks when young (Tebbich et al., 2010). However, developmental studies of tool use by New Caledonian crows suggest that much of their problem-solving skill involves both trial-and-error and social learning from watching what a parent or human tutor does (Holzhaider, Hunt & Gray, 2010; Kenward et al., 2006).

Another possibility, often raised in discussions of novel behaviour, is that the individual generalises from experience that it has obtained in other contexts (Shettleworth, 2010). Evidence that this can happen came from an experimental study in which pigeons were trained in the individual elements of behaviour that would eventually lead them, apparently 'insightfully', to push a box under a banana that was out of reach (Epstein et al., 1984). First, the pigeons were rewarded with grain for climbing onto a box and pecking a banana-like object. Jumping at the banana was not rewarded. The pigeons were then rewarded in interspersed trials for pushing the box to a place marked by a spot. Finally, they were tested with the banana out of reach but with the box not beneath it. After some conflict between looking up at the banana and looking at the box, the pigeons pushed the box around and, when it was under the banana, hopped onto it and pecked at the banana. In the final stage of the process, the pigeons behaved very much like Köhler's chimpanzees, but did this by generalising from the skills they had previously acquired through the sequence of training. This ability to put past experience to a new use might be regarded as a limited form of creativity.

A related possibility, which lies at the heart of this book, is that in the course of playing earlier in their lives, individuals discover properties of their environment that prove crucial when they are later faced with a new challenge. Young rooks, jays and magpies are playful, actively manipulating objects in ways that could reveal much about how the world works and what leads to what. They certainly pick up small stones and may even drop them into puddles, raising the level of the water. Similarly, young chimps readily play with sticks, and if they have played with bamboo sticks they might discover that a smaller stick can be threaded inside the hole of a larger one, creating a longer stick. This possibility was supported by one small-scale experiment showing that a chimp that had prior opportunities to play with sticks solved the problem, whereas individuals that had no such prior opportunities failed (Birch, 1945).

Perhaps the bubble-blowing humpback whales had at some point in the past discovered this remarkable hunting technique by playfully blowing bubbles and learning that fish will not swim through a bubble screen. Then perhaps they cooperated to create a cylindrical screen and drive the fish upwards to the surface where they could be caught easily. It is known that their playful relatives, the dolphins, do invent novel forms of behaviour and readily copy the novel behaviour of other dolphins. A similar process of discovery through play may plausibly have given rise to the remarkable feeding techniques of the humpbacks. Either way, the behaviour of these highly intelligent animals could reasonably be regarded as creative, because it involves the generation of new forms, and innovative, because the novel behaviour is then used for practical benefit and adopted by others.[18]

CONCLUSIONS

Some birds and some mammals have an astonishing ability to solve difficult problems in apparently insightful ways. The developmental processes that give rise to such remarkable cognitive abilities are not yet well understood. In some cases, playing earlier in life may have been involved in acquiring the necessary cognitive tools. The behaviour of dolphins and whales provides compelling examples of what appear to be creativity and innovation, some of which may have been facilitated by previous play.

7

People and organisations

We have argued from biological evidence that experiences gained during play can be used later in life and put together in novel ways to solve new problems. Play experiences may also lead immediately to the discovery of new ways of doing things. At the heart of play is the pleasure of engaging in the activity or thought process for its own sake, without any extrinsic reward. Even so, the creativity fostered by play can bring its own rewards. These will be intrinsic, but the rewards may also be material if creativity leads to successful innovation that benefits the player and others. In this chapter we first examine how others have viewed the satisfaction that creativity brings and the conditions that are conducive to creativity in organisations. We then consider how prior opportunities for play can facilitate the discovery of new ideas. Once discovered, the process of translating new ideas into innovations involves different skills.

INDIVIDUAL CREATIVITY

The social psychologist and educationalist Graham Wallas (1926) described five stages of the creative process, from preparation, incubation, intimation and illumination through to verification. Preparation involves formulating the problem to be solved. Incubation involves pondering potential solutions, possibly over a long period of time. Intimation involves articulating ways in which the problem might be solved, and illumination and verification involve testing the possibilities. Like others before him, Wallas considered creativity to be a process that allows humans to adapt to their changing environment. Since his time, the concept of creativity has developed extensively.

In Chapter 5 we described how creative people tend to be more open to new experiences, less conventional, less conscientious and more impulsive than less creative people. These characteristics are linked to relatively stable features of personality. Stability is often equated with inherited characteristics, but the notion that personality in some sense develops independently of experience is, to say the least, arguable. Clearly, experience has a great effect on behaviour and personality, particularly early in development (Bateson & Martin, 1999). The extent to which a child is playful depends on how he or she developed. For example, Barnett and Kleiber (1984) found that first-born boys were less playful than later-born ones, and other environmental factors such as the socioeconomic status of the family were also associated with differences in the children's playfulness.[19] The overall conclusion from a range of evidence is that environmental and epigenetic factors are likely to influence both playfulness and creativity.

Creativity is responsive to experience and can be influenced by specific forms of education. Training courses to enhance creativity in adults have been established and have had some degree of success, particularly in the domain of innovation. A meta-analysis of 70 published studies indicated that the more effective programmes focused on the development of cognitive skills and the application of those skills to specific problems (Scott, Leritz & Mumford, 2004). Simple practical measures can also help. Mihaly Csikszentmihalyi (1996) noted that a number of obstacles often lie in the path of personal creativity: exhaustion from too many demands, distractions that fragment thought, lack of direction and plain laziness can all get in the way of being creative. He argued that all of these barriers could be overcome, and offered advice on how to do it. The first step, he suggested, is to free up time from the pursuit of predictable goals in order to engage curiosity and look for surprises. With mental energy enhanced, Csikszentmihalyi recommended avoiding time-wasting distractions such as aimlessly watching television, and also making best use of the body's natural circadian rhythms, since most people are more productive at certain times of the day. He also suggested finding particular spaces and places that enhance reflective thought and creativity.

One especially important factor that is known to make a significant difference to creativity is the range and variety of contacts the individual has. Someone with just a few very familiar friends may lack stimulation and exposure to new ideas, whereas someone with a huge number of casual acquaintances may be overloaded. Around 50 people has been suggested as being about the optimal size of a personal network in order to stimulate creativity (King, 2012), although the nature and mix of those contacts is bound to be important. The use of social media enables interactions with much bigger networks and a much more extensive interchange of ideas. We believe that the degree of playfulness in the interactions someone has with their contacts may be a major influence on how creative they are. This issue relates to the creativity found in groups, which we consider in the next section.

As we argued in the Chapter 5, mood is crucial. Many authors have noted how a generally positive state of mind can stimulate creativity (e.g. Isen & Reeve, 2005; Lyubomirsky et al., 2005). We have argued that a particular kind of positive mood – the one associated with playfulness – may be especially beneficial. Playfulness, however, is not the only mood to affect creativity, and even negative moods may act as a stimulus. An individual who is indignant about some wrongdoing, for example, may be motivated to produce creative solutions to such a challenge. Emergencies, whether personal or national, can be a spur to major discovery such as the cracking of codes or the invention of new weapons during times of war. For some people, the prospect of large financial rewards can provide a powerful incentive to be creative and to turn the creative idea into a successful innovation.

Mood affects different aspects of creativity in different ways. Three dimensions of creativity, as described previously, are fluency, flexibility and originality. The evidence suggests that these facets of creativity are differentially affected by emotional state. A meta-analysis of the results of 102 separate studies showed how mood is associated with different aspects of creativity (Baas, De Dreu & Nijstad, 2008). Positive moods were found to produce more originality and fluency than negative moods, but they were not linked to other measures of creativity. However, the relationship between mood and creativity cannot be understood in terms of a simple dichotomy between positive and negative moods. So-called activating positive moods, such as elation, were found to be associated with higher levels of creativity, whereas deactivating positive moods, such as serenity, were not. This finding ran counter to the common belief that creative ideas emerge when people are relaxing. Furthermore, Baas et al. (2008) found suggestive evidence that some mood states, such as feeling happy, may generate original ideas through enhanced fluency, whereas others, such as anger, may exert their effects through enhanced persistence with the task. This difference makes sense in terms of the distinction we have drawn between generating new ideas (creativity) and turning those ideas into practical solutions that are adopted by others (innovation). Being a successful innovator is likely to require many psychological and emotional attributes – such as determination, focus and resilience – that may have little to do with the ability to generate novel thoughts.

CREATIVITY IN GROUPS

A much-used approach in encouraging people to be creative is to bring them together in groups, whether physically or virtually, using social media. Many more opportunities for combining disparate thoughts in creative ways will arise when people interact with each other rather than working in isolation. And indeed, the evidence shows that groups or networks are generally much more successful at consistently producing useful new ideas than solitary individuals. For example, the analysis by Steven Johnson (2010), which we mentioned in Chapter 5, found that two-thirds of successful ideas had come from networks rather than single individuals. The most creative and inventive organisations, such as Google, Apple, MIT Media Lab and Bell Labs, have recognised this and have put in place institutional mechanisms intended specifically to bring together people from different backgrounds in order to maximise the intermingling of disparate ideas.

An important ingredient for success in creative group endeavours is for the group to contain people with a wide range of knowledge and skills. Diversity encourages greater creativity, and multidisciplinary approaches are of proven effectiveness in generating new ideas (e.g. Alves et al., 2007). The diversity of the participants increases the likelihood that novel combinations of ideas and experience will be brought together. Many of these novel combinations will not result in good ideas, but the chances of success are improved. As well as diverse knowledge, creative groups also benefit from having a preference for thinking in novel ways, persistence in overcoming obstacles, and a willingness to have fun (Sternberg, O'Hara & Lubart, 1997).

The value of bringing people together lies behind many common techniques for producing ideas. Recognising that people are not always good at devising arresting new ideas when working on their own, an advertising executive called Alex Osborn (1952) encouraged his colleagues to work in groups in order to 'brainstorm', as he called it. He suggested that brainstorming groups should follow four simple rules.

1. They should focus on *quantity* of ideas, since this increases the chances of coming up with an idea of real quality. In terms of creativity, this means maximising fluency rather than originality or flexibility.
2. The participants should withhold all criticism.
3. They should actively welcome unusual ideas.
4. They should be encouraged to combine unusual ideas to generate something even more imaginative.

When the brainstorming process worked well, social inhibitions broke down and, it was argued, imaginative ideas flowed freely.

The basic idea of brainstorming has long since entered the public consciousness and is still widely regarded as a standard way of generating ideas. However, the effectiveness of brainstorming, as it is often practised, has been called into doubt by evidence suggesting that it may in fact not work as well as it is supposed to. In one meta-analysis, Diehl and Stroebe (1991) found that in 18 out of the 22 published studies they examined, groups of people brainstorming together actually produced *fewer* original ideas than individuals working separately or in groups that discussed ideas in more conventional ways. Moreover, members of brainstorming groups often overestimated the value of their inventiveness and fell into the trap of supposing they had come up with a particularly good idea.

One reason why simple brainstorming often falls short is because it fails to follow its own rules of creating a truly protected context in which new ideas can be offered without fear of criticism. In practice, dominant members of the group may hog the discussion and inhibit others who do not want to make fools of themselves. Moreover, the activity of some members encourages laziness in others, who do not exert themselves and therefore contribute less. As a result, potentially fruitful avenues may not be explored. In contrast, a well-conducted conventional group discussion, in which everyone is permitted to analyse and criticise new ideas, may encourage all the participants to work harder, think more deeply, and therefore contribute more to the quantity and quality of ideas. Empirical evidence indicates that debate and productive criticism may actually stimulate good ideas rather than inhibiting them (Nemeth et al., 2004). Again, the parallel with play is worth noting: play occurs in a protected context without concern for the outcome, and the positive mood associated with playfulness may encourage divergent thinking.[20]

A common feature of the most creative and innovative organisations is that employees are less subject to heavy bureaucratic constraints. Those responsible for generating the new ideas are often allowed free time to think laterally and explore wild ideas, without being punished for wasting time. The 3M Company, for example, encourages people to devote time, known as the 'boot-legging hour', to activities that at first sight might seem unproductive (Lehrer, 2012). The company allows every researcher to spend 15% of their working day pursuing speculative ideas. Using a similar principle, Google gives its software engineers the freedom of what it calls 'innovation time off'. The free flow of ideas is encouraged throughout the day and canteens, where people can meet to talk, provide free food. Other innovative companies such as Netflix have removed most of the administrative burdens from its potentially creative employees in order to develop a productive environment. Organisations that rely on innovation must also be willing to risk more failures in the initial creative stages (Kanter, 2006). The effectiveness of such approaches will of course depend on the nature of the company, and raw creativity may be less critical in retail or service industries than it is in, say, technology sectors that depend for their survival on sustaining rapid innovation. But in almost any workplace, creativity is more likely to thrive when employees are given some freedom to develop their own ideas and interact playfully with others (Scott & Bruce, 1994).

Working conditions can clearly facilitate or impede creativity (Amabile et al., 1996). While less research attention has been directed to environments that impede creativity, a number of factors distinguish between high-creativity environments and those associated with low creativity. People working in a highly creative environment tend to receive more encouragement by the parent organisation and the supervisors of projects. More freedom and resources are given to those working on new projects. By providing a more relaxed working atmosphere, the intrinsic motivation of those involved in generating creative solutions can be enhanced (McLean, 2005).

A limited amount of empirical research has been conducted on the design of physical environments conducive to creativity (Moultrie et al., 2007). It suggests that factors such as the colour of the surroundings may have some influence on mood and creativity. In one study, people were more creative in response to test questions about alternative uses presented to them on a computer when the background screen colour was blue (Mehta & Zhu, 2009). This lends support to the belief that creativity can be mildly stimulated by painting walls blue. Some indirect evidence about the subtle influence of the physical environment comes from research on the design of hospitals. One study found that patients in hospital wards in which they could see trees outside recovered more quickly after surgery and required fewer analgesics than patients who could not see outside (Ulrich, 1984). Subsequent research found that nursing staff were more likely to stay in their jobs if they worked in hospital wards with outside views. Everybody, it seemed, was a little bit happier and a little less stressed. An academic journal called *Health, Environments, Research and Design (HERD)* is devoted to evidence-based designs intended to improve health (e.g. Ulrich et al., 2010). Given the importance of positive mood to playfulness and creativity, it seems likely that the type of research published in *HERD* could also be useful in designing environments that are conducive to generating novel and interesting ideas. The ideal environment might be one that helps to foster the right balance of social interaction, stimulation and playfulness without being excessively relaxing. Creativity cannot be forced, but it can be encouraged.

THE ROLE OF PLAY AND PLAYFULNESS

In their book *Sparks of Genius*, Robert and Michèle Root-Bernstein (2001) explored the playfulness of famous scientists, artists and composers. In describing their work, creative people often make passing reference to a positive or playful mood and to toying with ideas. Other academics, such as Sternberg, O'Hara and Lubart (1997), have been explicit about the importance for creativity of having fun. In the foregoing discussion of creativity, many of the conditions that enhance the generation of new ideas are precisely those generated by play and, in particular, by playful play, in which play is accompanied by a positive, light-hearted mood that fosters divergent thinking and the connection of previously unconnected thoughts. Positive social interactions are potentially important in generating the right mood. So too is freedom from burdensome constraints and the availability of a stress-free (but not excessively relaxing) environment. Intrinsic motivation and fluency of thought are enhanced when curiosity is aroused and the individual is looking for surprises. Immediate success or failure are irrelevant to the activity, at least while it is in progress. The essence of play involves entering many blind alleys that often lead nowhere but occasionally lead somewhere really interesting.

Although creativity and innovation are often used interchangeably in the context of business, we have distinguished between them. We framed creativity in terms of the generation of novel ideas, whereas innovation is the successful implementation of those ideas and their uptake by others. Creativity, in this sense, is a necessary precursor to innovation, providing the raw material for a successful outcome. While we think a strong case can be made for the role of play and playfulness in fostering creativity, the successful implementation and spread of a good idea requires many further steps and different skills, including persistence, analytical thinking and attention to detail. Play and playfulness are more directly relevant to creativity (in our terms) than they are to innovation.

INNOVATION

The crucial importance of creativity and innovation to organisations and nations should be self-evident. The most successful companies take active steps to foster the creation of new ideas and see them through to implementation. However, some organisations and companies, often the less successful ones, do little more than pay lip service to the principle (Kanter, 2009). With that possibly in mind, President Obama stressed the importance of creativity and innovation in his 2011 State of the Union message:

> The first step in winning the future is encouraging American innovation. None of us can predict with certainty what the next big industry will be or where the new jobs will come from. Thirty years ago, we couldn't know that something called the Internet would lead to an economic revolution. What we can do – what America does better than anyone else – is spark the creativity and imagination of our people. We're the nation that put cars in driveways and computers in offices; the nation of Edison and the Wright brothers; of Google and Facebook. In America, innovation doesn't just change our lives. It is how we make our living.

When creativity gives rise to innovation, the winnowing of new ideas, as described by Campbell (1960) and others, becomes central. Many ideas, including some cherished ones, may have to be discarded. The process of converting a creative idea into a successful innovation can involve extremely hard and pro- longed work and may not be at all playful. The discoverers of the molecular structure of DNA, Jim Watson and Francis Crick, were highly competitive with their potential rivals and always eager to beat them to uncovering what they referred to as the secret of life.

Although playful creativity is often an essential precursor to successful innovation, it may sometimes cause tensions within organisations, particularly those under intense commer- cial pressure. At worst, a degree of conflict may arise between those who are given considerable freedom to play with interest- ing new concepts and those responsible for transforming those concepts as rapidly and cheaply as possible into practical, revenue-earning products (Kanter, 2006). Leadership and man- agerial skills may be required to avoid such conflict. Managers overseeing the innovative process must also keep an eye on potentially destructive criticism or scepticism, just as they do at the initial stage of generating creative ideas. The general manager of invention factory IDEO noted that a new idea or proposal can be buried when somebody says: 'Let me just play devil's advocate for a minute'. Having invoked the protective power of that phrase, the critic can easily destroy the fledgling concept (Kelley, 2006). The positive and cooperative mood that is so important in fostering creativity serves an important role at the implementation stage as well.

Creativity, and hence innovation, may be improved simply by doing more, and thereby creating more potential opportuni- ties for new ideas to succeed. One piece of empirical evidence that supports this principle is the correlation that exists between the *quality* of music, literature or science produced by individuals and the *quantity* of work they have previously produced for public consumption (Simonton, 1997). Productivity in the arts and the sciences tends to grow with experience, although the peak in quality tends to come early in fields such as mathematics.

Andrew Hargadon and Robert Sutton (2000) spent 5 years studying innovative businesses and concluded that success has little to do with nurturing solitary genius and everything to do with organisation and attitude. As they put it, the best innovators 'serve as intermediaries, or brokers, between otherwise disconnected pools of ideas. They use their in-between vantage point to spot old ideas that can be used in new places, new ways, and new combinations.' The process involves capturing good ideas, keeping ideas alive, imagining new uses for old ideas, and putting promising concepts to the test. Keeping ideas alive is important where valuable information may otherwise be lost when employees move on. To safeguard against such losses, some companies store ideas in collections of electronic records, notes, drawings and even – in some cases – discarded material that may look like junk but could embody potentially interesting ideas. According to Hargadon and Sutton, the most respected innovators have large private collections of stuff, know where to find things, and go out of their way to help others by sharing their knowledge. So-called invention factories, which specialise in providing innovative solutions for other organisations, collect related products and writings on those products, and take time to observe users of existing products.

As we have already pointed out, excellence in one area of activity, such as creativity, is not necessarily accompanied by excellence in another area such as practical innovation. The creative people who came up with the ideas are not always the best equipped for testing and putting them into practice. The different skills involved in producing ideas and turning them into reality are reflected in a lack of correlation between creativity in early life and material success in later life (Runco et al., 2010). But even if creativity is not a certain road to riches, the creative people in that study stated, towards the end of their lives, that they had gained considerable personal satisfaction from what they had done.

The academic study of innovation has grown massively in the past half century.[21] In his introduction to the *Oxford Handbook of Innovation*, Fagerberg (2005) noted that invention, in the sense of coming up with a good creative idea, and innovation are so closely linked that they are hard to distinguish from each other, as in biotechnology, for example; but that a considerable time lag often occurs between the two. Even when a creative idea has been transformed into a working product, it may still fail to corner the market in the face of competition, costs, production difficulties or consumer indifference. Time and again, transformational technological innovations have been preceded by other innovations that encapsulated the basic creative ideas but failed to take off commercially. For example, the MP3 player arrived before the iPod and simple personal computers preceded the IBM PC and Apple Macintosh. Good ideas can be around for a long time before they become commercially successful products. As in the case of play behaviour in young organisms, the benefits may not accrue until much later. Commercial or artistic products that are judged to be innovative must be original. At the same time, however, the successful innovator must not produce work that is excessively novel, because it may seem disagreeably strange to others.

CONCLUSIONS

Facilitating play and playfulness can be helpful in generating new ideas that in turn may become new products or new ways of doing things. For the individual, the experiences accumulated during play may not be useful immediately – though some may. However, they may be of great significance later on, when the individual is faced with a challenge that requires a creative solution. In organisations concerned with making new discoveries, the practical implementation of new ideas generally requires different skills from those needed for generating the ideas in the first place.

8

Childhood play and creativity

Even the most cursory glance at humanity reveals the enormous importance of each person's experience, upbringing and culture. Take the astonishing variation among humans in language, dietary habits, mating customs, child-care practices, clothing, religion, architecture, art, and much else besides. Nobody could seriously doubt the remarkable human capacity for learning from personal experience and learning from others. Many of the differences between people derive from what happened to them when they were young. It would be very surprising, therefore, if play in childhood had no effect on adult behaviour. The question that is central to the theme of this book is this: does play in childhood enhance creativity in later life? Governments of all stripes recognise the need for innovation in order to produce prosperity. Scientists and engineers similarly understand the need for creative and innovative thinkers in their profession. We argue in this chapter that play and playfulness in childhood are potentially important in making adults more creative. Play comes in many forms, particularly in children, so we consider whether some types of play are more important than others in affecting subsequent creativity. We also touch on the role of playfulness in education.[22]

The belief that play is an important part of how children acquire knowledge has been extraordinarily influential in educational circles in Britain and North America. Peter Smith (2010) commented that many researchers in this field had gone too far in assuming that play was essential for normal development and that playing was the best, or only, way of acquiring essential skills and experience. Such scepticism about the significance of play has not removed concern on the part of others that apparent restrictions on aspects of children's play in the developed world could have unfortunate and unintended consequences for their development. We return to this issue later in the chapter.

PLAY, PLAYFULNESS AND CREATIVITY

We noted in Chapter 5 how creative scientists, composers and artists are often described as being playful in their professional activities. Many of the MacArthur Fellows who were honoured for their creative work as adults reported engaging in extensive imaginary play during their childhood and regarded their play as having relevance for their adult work (Root-Bernstein & Root-Bernstein, 2006). As one of the scientists said: 'It is necessary to imagine what needs to be discovered before discovery can be made'. Such evidence is merely suggestive rather than conclusive, because a comparison group was lacking and the study was retrospective. In contrast to the MacArthur Fellows, when the Root-Bernsteins asked college science students about the importance of their childhood play, the students failed to see its relevance to their scientific careers. The Root-Bernsteins speculated that many science students are not encouraged to value the imaginative or playful aspects of their discipline and underestimate the creativity needed to succeed in it. Science students often have so much material to assimilate that they have little opportunity to think creatively.

The question of whether play and playfulness lead to creativity, the other way round, or both facilitate each other, has proved difficult to answer. In an early study, girls and boys who played more were more creative in terms of their originality and fluency than a matched control sample of children who played less (Torrance, 1961).[23] Evidence that playfulness (as distinct from play) is linked to creativity came from research by Nina Lieberman (1977). She defined playfulness as a state in which the child exhibits spontaneity, manifest joy and a sense of humour. Playful, friendly teasing was distinguished from hostile wit, which is not playful. Lieberman found that the more playful children were also more creative. What might be responsible for such differences in creativity? One hypothesis is that playfulness boosts creativity. Another is that a predisposition to being creative could also enhance playfulness. Studies such as those of Lieberman and others that followed raised important questions about the causal link between play, playfulness and creativity, but were unable to answer them.

In order to study causality, an experimental approach is required. Many experiments have attempted to give some children more opportunities to play while other children, acting as a comparison group, have not experienced this intervention. The results have not always matched expectations. In one study, Moore and Rudd (2008) studied the effects of play on creativity 2–8 months after a play intervention. Forty-five children aged 6–8 years participated in five 30-minute individual sessions over a period of 3–5 weeks. They were randomly assigned to one of three groups. In the first group, each child was asked to make up their own stories about specified topics. Children in the second group were encouraged to express their feelings when given a set of toys, including dolls, blocks, plastic animals, Lego toys and cars. Members of the third group, initially classified as the controls, were asked to put together puzzles and colour pictures in a book. When the children were subsequently assessed using tests of alternative uses, the supposed control group unexpectedly scored the highest of the three groups on measures of creative thinking. The authors speculated that some unknown aspects of the play intervention might have interfered with the creative processes of the children in the other two groups. For example, attempting to fit a story into an ordered and logical structure might have inhibited mental flexibility and the generation of multiple associations. Moreover, some aspects of the 'control' procedure might have inadvertently facilitated the children's creativity, perhaps because they were not constrained by specific storylines. Even though the adults supervising the experiment attempted to limit discussion to standardised prompts, the children in the 'control' group were free to talk about events in their daily lives and think about whatever they wanted. Whatever the actual reasons, these findings emphasise how subtle the effects of play interventions can be.

In an important experimental study of play and creativity, 86 Spanish children aged 10 and 11 years were initially assessed for their verbal and graphic creativity (Garaigordobil, 2006). The subsequent play interventions consisted of a 2-hour play session once a week for most of the school year. In each session the children were told about the aims of each game and were given instructions for carrying it out. One of the games involved each player receiving a sheet of paper and a pencil, dividing the sheet in half by drawing a line across the centre, and then drawing an animal in the upper half. When the player had finished the drawing, he or she passed it to the player on one side and received another sheet from the player on the other. The second player then had to draw another animal in the lower half of the sheet, incorporating a part of the body from the animal in the upper half. The transformation was then described by the second child at the bottom of the sheet. So, for example, the first child might have drawn an elephant and his or her partner might have drawn a butterfly, using the ears of the elephant as wings. The second child might then describe the finished drawing as 'the elephant has turned into a butterfly'. Other games included inventing advertisements for a product or service; drawing, as a team, a mural on a large sheet of paper; inventing new names for familiar objects; devising funny drawings; and conducting imaginary conversations over the telephone. After the game, the children sat in a circle and each team presented its conclusions about what its members had done. This was followed by a discussion in which the results of their activities were analysed. Children in a control group carried out supervised artistic activities from the normal school curriculum, receiving the same overall level of attention from adults as those in the play intervention group.

At the end of the school year, the children were all tested for their ability to produce new ideas (fluency), their aptitude for changing from one line of thought to another (flexibility), and their capacity to find solutions that were far from obvious, common, or established (originality). In testing originality, for example, the child was presented with a black blot and asked to draw something that included the blot and give the drawing a title. The children were also asked to paint a picture on a theme of their own choice. Their paintings were judged independently by artists, who were asked to look for, among other things, novelty, fantasy and breaking away from reality.

The results revealed a clear link between the children's play experience and their subsequent creativity. The boys and girls who received more opportunities for play significantly increased their verbal and graphic creativity scores compared with the controls. The biggest effects of the additional play experience were seen in those children who had scored low on creativity before the intervention.[24] These results are all the more compelling because considerable efforts were made to control for other aspects of the intervention that were not directly related to play experience. The intermittent intervention extended over most of the school year, so the results cannot be explained by a short-term boost in playfulness or general activity. We think this study provides good evidence that the play experiences of the children in the intervention group boosted their creativity at a later stage,[25] although it did not show whether the effects persisted into later life. This could be a goal for future research.

PRETEND PLAY

Pretend play by children imitates adult actions in a non-functional context, such as playing at being a doctor. Pretend play may not be playful in the sense that we have defined it, involving a positive and light-hearted mood. Moreover it may not result in greater creativity on the part of the child. A thorough and critical review of the influence of pretend play on a variety of cognitive dimensions in children, including creativity, concluded that pretend play has little measurable effect (Lillard et al., 2013). The authors considered three hypotheses that had originally been proposed by Peter Smith (2010); namely, that pretend play has a direct causal influence on cognition; or it is one of several processes that can lead to the same endpoint (equifinality); or that pretend play is a side-effect or epiphenomenon of other processes involved in the development of cognition. They concluded that the evidence for pretend play enhancing creativity is not convincing, and argued that the occurrence of pretend play is correlated with some other, unspecified, factor that relates to creativity. Lillard et al. (2013) commented that the studies they reviewed were limited in many ways and more high-quality research was needed. Sample sizes were often very small, the play interventions were often very limited in scale, and the measurements of creativity were often questionable.

Despite this negative conclusion that pretend play does not appear to boost creativity, at least when measured in standard ways, some long-term changes in pretend play are interesting. One study examined trends over a 23-year period in pretend play among 6–10-year-old children (Russ & Dillon, 2011). The results showed that the level of imagination exhibited in children's play increased significantly over the period, even though the children had less time to play. Whether or not this change over time was associated with greater creativity was not clear.

OTHER EFFECTS OF PLAY

In addition to fostering creativity, play can also enhance children's cognitive ability. The role of play in problem-solving was studied in 3–5-year-old children (Sylva, Bruner & Genova, 1976). The children were given opportunities to play with sticks and clamps and were subsequently asked to retrieve a desirable object (a piece of coloured chalk) that was placed too far away to be reached by hand. They were compared with a group of children who had observed adults clamping sticks together and a group that had no experience of playing with the objects or seeing adults doing it. The results showed that playing with the objects, or watching adults using them, affected the children's problem-solving. Significantly more children in the group that had played spontaneously with the objects learned to solve the problem, compared with the no-treatment group. Children in the play group did not differ from the children who had been shown the principle by adults, but their problem-solving method was different. The children who had played with the objects initially tried to reach the chalk with one stick and, after failing, they clamped the sticks together to make a longer stick that enabled them to retrieve the chalk. In contrast, the group that had only watched the adults solve the problem were less systematic and more inflexible in their problem-solving. In addition, the children who had played with the objects were more motivated than the children in the two comparison groups and less frustrated by failure. The evidence suggests that playing can improve aspects of children's problem-solving and motivation, at least in the short term.

A meta-analysis of 46 published studies found that the amount that children played was correlated with their skills in language and cognition and their relationships with other people (Fisher, 1992). Especially clear links with cognitive and social abilities were found for play involving the acting-out of scenes from cartoons or books, in which the children adopted roles or gave roles to dolls or puppets. Suggestive though this evidence is, the causal link between play and other behavioural characteristics was not established. Many other factors, such as the home environment, could have independently affected both playfulness and cognitive development.

PLAYFULNESS AND EDUCATION

Children may learn directly through play. But play and playfulness can also contribute indirectly to more conventional forms of learning. Academic achievement may be fostered by motivating pupils through a variety of activities that introduce an element of play into what might otherwise be regarded as 'serious' work. The value of creating a playful learning environment is increasingly emphasised by many writers (e.g. Bergen, 2009; Kangas, 2010). Asian educationalists who are concerned about the excessive formality of school teaching have been moving in this direction. Others in the West have capitalised on pupils' familiarity with social media and computer games to help them compose more imaginative work (Colby & Colby, 2008). Students have been encouraged to move from small-scale personal projects to large-scale projects by working play-fully with others in a virtual world. Although the use of such approaches to enhance creativity seems intuitively the right way to go, judgement about the academic and social benefits must await further research.

In contrast to the use of playful approaches in education, concerns have been expressed about children spending too much time watching videos and television, often at the expense of playing socially or physically. A study of 400 stories written by 36 children aged 10–12 years concluded that watching television and videos is more likely to stifle than to stimulate children's imagination (Belton, 2001). Teresa Belton recognised that tele-vision does have the potential to stimulate children's imaginative thinking, and she provided good examples of where it had done so. The potential was seldom realised, however. The children's own direct experience proved more salient for their story-making. It seems that bombardment with mediated images and ideas robs children of the opportunity to devise their own activ-ities and develop their own thought processes – which is often best done through play. The more general point about playful approaches to education was made strongly in a report by the UK Parliamentary Office of Science and Technology (POST, 2000). It concluded that well-resourced pre-schools that encourage the development of emotional, cognitive and social skills and feelings of self-efficacy, through natural activities such as play and exploration, result in lasting social and educational benefits. The benefits are especially valuable for children from deprived backgrounds.

SENSITIVE PERIODS

Particular skills or types of knowledge tend to be acquired most readily at particular stages in development. A familiar example of a sensitive period for learning is the development of lan-guage. Children who have been massively deprived of social contact and then rescued show remarkable resilience, and yet the difficulty of learning language at a later age than normal often proves one of their greatest stumbling blocks. An accent derived from childhood experience is particularly difficult to lose in a newly acquired second language, and some vowel and consonant sounds in the new language may not be recognised at all (Bateson & Martin, 1999). A number of important conclusions have emerged from studies of sensitive periods for learning. The developmental processes that make learning easier at the beginning of a sensitive period are often linked to the stage of the child's development. This point has relevance for the timing of children's education, where earlier does not necessarily mean better.

There is no convincing evidence to suggest that teaching children reading, writing and mathematics before about the age of 6 years is advantageous (POST, 2000). The POST report argued that a slightly later school starting age of 6 or 7 years might be preferable, provided that it was preceded by high-quality pre-school provision. Nonetheless, an emphasis on acquiring the 3Rs (reading, 'riting and 'rithmetic) at an early age is increasingly common in the UK (Anning, 2010). Children in the UK are placed in a classroom regime at an earlier age than is usual in other European countries, although formal teaching starts early in China. Do children benefit in the long run from starting schooling at the age of four? The educationalist Janet Moyles (2010) argued forcefully that they do not. Indeed, some evidence suggests that teaching these skills at too early an age may increase children's anxiety and diminish their motivation to learn (Elkind, 2008).

As in all prescriptions, one size does not fit all. Some children develop much more rapidly than others and educational practices should be sufficiently flexible to allow for such differences. In her review of the early years foundations for life, health and learning in the UK, Clare Tickell (2012) recommended that the bureaucratic rules should be made much less burdensome in order to encourage greater flexibility, and the formal targets for early years education should be reduced fourfold. Among other things, she also recommended that play should be recognised as an important part of teaching and learning, reinforcing what had been emphasised in a much earlier report by Bridget Plowden (1967).

A growing concern expressed by many writers in economically developed countries is that children may be disadvantaged by being deprived of opportunities for certain forms of play experience (Palmer, 2006; Ward, 2012). Doubtless it was commonplace for children in earlier centuries, or currently in impoverished parts of the world, to be deprived of play, but in more affluent times or nations it is feared that opportunities for play are diminishing.

These concerns about a decline in play are supported by a considerable body of empirical evidence. When contemporary children's experiences of outdoor play in the UK were compared with their parents' accounts of their own childhood, the children were found to play much less outdoors and were much more likely to play in their homes (Valentine & McKendrick, 1997). In a similar study in the USA, 830 mothers nationwide were asked about their own play experiences as children, as well as their children's play experiences (Clements, 2004). The children were reported to spend considerably less time playing outdoors than their mothers had done as children. Even allowing for distortions in parental memories of an imagined golden childhood, the evidence for a decline in the opportunity to play freely outside is strong (Gleave, 2009). The most significant influences on children's access to independent play are parental anxieties about safety, and dependence on television and digital media, rather than the provision of public play facilities. Parental anxieties about safety and time spent watching TV are themselves connected, as shown by another study in which children who lived in neighbourhoods that were perceived by their mothers as unsafe were found to watch more television (Burdette & Whitaker, 2005).

Parental concerns about children's security have led to changes in the nature of childhood, with unintended consequences. The tendency of some parents to misjudge risks and overprotect their offspring from all sorts of real and largely imagined dangers may have adverse implications for their children's psychological and physical well-being (Furedi, 2001; Martin, 2005; Murrin & Martin, 2004). Once-common activities such as roaming freely with friends, or even walking unescorted to and from school, are becoming increasingly rare experiences for young children in the UK. It is widely believed that children should not be left on their own outside, and the activities of many children are closely monitored to ensure they do not come to harm. Alternatively, they are encouraged to stay at home. The unintended consequences can include having fewer opportunities to learn how to interact effectively with other children, deal with aggression, cross busy roads, function independently, or manage everyday risks. Depriving children of opportunities for free play also deprives them of opportunities for physical exercise, making them more susceptible to becoming obese and unfit.

To make matters worse, the time available for free play in schools has also been steadily eroding (Blatchford & Baines, 2006; Pellegrini, 2009). Stricter codes about safety have rendered school playgrounds less physically challenging and interesting (Copeland et al., 2012). Financial constraints may limit a school's ability to install the best playground equipment. Some parents, concerned about potential injury or upset from rough-and-tumble play, have even requested school staff to restrict their children's playground activities. Furthermore, those with responsibility for pre-school children feel pressure from parents to provide more structured teaching at the expense of opportunities for unstructured play. Scheduled playtime is increasingly squeezed by the pressures of an expanding curriculum, competitive league tables and the demands of parents.

The reduction in breaks or recesses during the school day has many potentially adverse consequences for children (Blatchford & Baines, 2006). They have less opportunity to meet and play with their friends. This is even more important when children are less likely to meet after school because of parental concerns about safety or, in many cases, larger distances between schools and homes. Cutting down on free time may also be counterproductive from an educational standpoint, because children are unable to maintain their concentration for very long without a break.

Some writers have perceived particularly dire consequences from the reduction in children's experiences of playing freely outdoors with other children. For example, the psychologist Peter Gray (2011) has suggested that the decline in such experience could explain why anxiety, depression, suicide, feelings of helplessness, and narcissism have increased among children, adolescents and young adults. He has argued that play functions as the major means by which children develop intrinsic interests and competencies, learn how to make decisions, solve problems, exert self-control, learn to regulate their emotions, make friends, learn to get along with others as equals, and experience joy. Other authors have made similarly strong claims about the benefits of play and the loss to children from being deprived of it. For instance, Stuart Brown (2009) has argued that play stimulates the imagination and 'invigorates the soul', making life meaningful, fulfilling and worthwhile. Brown and other play enthusiasts may well be right, but the empirical evidence is rarely as strong as the assertions. What is striking, however, is how scores for creative thought have declined in recent years, as measured by the Torrance test (Kim, 2011). Analysis of the normative data for the USA from 1966 to 2008 showed that creative thinking scores remained static or decreased, starting at around 11–12 years of age. Since 1990, creative thinking scores have significantly decreased, with the biggest decline in children aged up to around 9 years. If opportunities for playfulness are linked to creativity, this trend indicates that those who are concerned about the advent of what Sue Palmer (2006) calls a toxic childhood are right to worry.

ALTERNATIVE WAYS OF DEVELOPING

Even if children are playing less or playing differently, compared with the past, they may compensate in other ways, as we suggested might be possible in Chapter 3. Alternative modes of development might lead to the same outcome in adulthood. Such a possibility would argue against the strong claims of some play enthusiasts. It would also bring comfort to the many parents who have good cause to worry about the safety of their children, given the increases in road traffic. Whatever the costs, they feel justified in restricting their children's freedom to roam. Their children might play beneficially inside their homes and interact playfully with their peers via social media. When they are not playing, children at home might gain intellectually from their access to the internet, social media, television and computer games. What they lose in one way, children might gain in another way. Average scores of IQ in many countries have tended to rise in the second half of the twentieth century (Flynn, 1987). The intelligence quotient or IQ is a measure of cognitive capacity. It is most strongly linked to analytical ability and a convergent mentality and not so strongly related to a creative divergent mentality.

Tempering the optimistic view that children find alternative forms of healthy development, some evidence suggests that the trend towards increased IQ has recently reversed in Western countries (Teasdale & Owen, 2008). At the same time, as we have already noted, a decrease in scores for creative thinking has also been reported (Kim, 2011). These discouraging recent trends have been interpreted in terms of changes in educational practice, particularly in the USA (Bronson & Merryman, 2010). Or they may result from decreased opportunities for free play. Whatever the explanation, the hoped-for benefits of an alternative experience of childhood do not seem to have materialised.

A different type of childhood is likely to lead to a different type of adult. Much has been made of the different styles of education in East Asia and the West (Kim, 2005). In Asia the emphasis has been on disciplined acquisition of knowledge. In the West, educational practices have been more conducive to enabling creativity, at least in the relatively recent past. But differences between East and West have been disappearing. As we have already noted, pressures on school curricula have contributed to fewer opportunities for play by children in the West. If our thesis is correct, then the loss of time for playing is likely to have contributed to the observed decline in creative thought.

CONCLUSIONS

Obtaining good evidence about the effects of childhood play on creativity is not easy. Devising control procedures for experimental play interventions is difficult, and guarding against the inadvertent favouring of children who receive more play experience requires special precautions. Nonetheless, the increasingly sophisticated research in this area suggests that some types of play do boost creativity. We are impressed by evidence of short-term links between play in childhood and creativity. Creativity, we believe, can be fostered by some aspects of play, particularly playful play. Some evidence suggests that these benefits may persist, although more research is needed.

The long-term effects of different types of childhood experience remain uncertain. But the overall picture suggests that those who determine the shape of education have much to gain from fostering a positive, playful mood in the learning environment. Playfulness can enhance children's motivation so that they remain interested in a task, rather than getting frustrated and giving up. The adverse consequences of reducing opportunities for physical play and unsupervised social play may include impaired physical fitness, obesity, reduced sociality and reduced creativity. Our focus has been on creativity, but children's experience of play is of course likely to affect other attributes, such as their ability to communicate and form successful relationships with other people. All these consequences of childhood play are, in turn, likely to affect the cognitive and social styles, and ultimate well-being, of adults.

9

Humour and playfulness

Humorous people often behave playfully and playful people tend to have a good sense of humour. At face value, play and humour are connected. Further consideration reveals some shared underlying features. Play and humour both occur in protected contexts, where the rules of engagement are somehow different from 'serious' behaviour. They are both intrinsically motivating and enjoyable for their own sake. They are both accompanied, at least in some instances, by a distinctive positive mood. And they both involve combining things in unusual ways. Like play, humour is associated with the generation of novel and occasionally fruitful ideas and therefore can be highly creative.

Charles Darwin (1877) saw the connection between humour and play when he kept careful notes on the development of his first child, William Erasmus. Like many parents before him and since, he found that the game of peek-a-boo generated great amusement and laughter-like gurgling in his child. He wrote: 'I was at first surprised at humour being appreciated by an infant only a little above three months old, but we should remember how very early puppies and kittens begin to play.' The educational psychologist Nina Lieberman (1977), who worked on creativity in schoolchildren, also saw a link between humour and playfulness. Indeed, she used humour as part of her definition of playfulness in the children she studied.

In yet another parallel with play, humour is notoriously difficult to define and has spawned a large and often speculative literature on its nature and function. The defining features of humour have been hard to pin down, in much the same way as biologists and psychologists have struggled to define play. Like play, humour comes in many different forms, such as puns, jokes, riddles, satire, farce, caricature, slapstick and cartoons. To add to the complexity, individuals and cultures differ in what they find funny, and some forms of humour may be specific to a particular time and place. Nonetheless, most humour does seem to have certain underlying features, such as the use of exaggeration or incongruity, in which ideas are suddenly juxtaposed in surprising ways. What, then, is the nature of the relationship between play, playfulness, humour and creativity?

JOKES

Jokes are a particular form of humour. They come in many different shapes and can be highly specific to a particular context. Whether or not a joke is funny depends on the social context and how it is told (Forabosco, 1992). What many jokes have in common, however, is an element of surprise or incongruity. They work because they involve ideas that run against expectations, often because of a mismatch between setting the scene and the resolution. The humour lies in the surprise generated by the punch line. Surprise alone is not sufficient; it may even be alarming. Rather, it is the juxtaposition of an expectation and a surprise that is relevant to that expectation. Here is an example that won a competition run by Richard Wiseman and the British Association for the Advancement of Science to find the world's most popular joke:

> Two hunters are out in the woods when one of them collapses. He doesn't seem to be breathing and his eyes are glazed. The other guy whips out his phone and calls the emergency services. He gasps, 'My friend is dead! What can I do?' The operator says 'Calm down. I can help. First, let's make sure he's dead.' There is a silence, then a shot is heard. Back on the phone, the guy says 'OK, now what?'[26]

The organisers of the competition commented that jokes sometimes make people feel superior to others, reduce the emotional impact of anxiety-provoking events, or surprise them. The hunter joke was thought to contain all three elements. The reader feels superior to the stupid hunter, appreciates the humour in his misunderstanding of the operator, and is surprised by the punch line. That said, the slightly feeble nature of the world's most popular joke may represent the lowest common denominator of people from widely differing backgrounds and cultures, as the organisers noted themselves.

WHAT GENERATES HUMOUR?

One long-established view about the nature of humour is that it involves bringing together ideas from widely differing contexts to produce a surprising and incongruous combination. The parallel with play is clear. As Arthur Koestler (1964) put it, humour results when two different frames of reference are set up and a collision is generated between them. Not all humour relies on surprise or incongruity, and some examples may amuse despite having been repeated many times. Even so, much humour does result from the unexpected relevance of a surprising combination – the detection of incongruity followed by its resolution. The concept of incongruity refers to the relationship between the components of an object, event, idea, social expectation, and so forth. When the arrangement of the components is incompatible with the normal or expected pattern, the situation is perceived as incongruous (McGee, 1979). The hypothesis here is that people find funny the things that surprise them because they seem out of place: they leap to an interpretation on the basis of previous experience that is shown by subsequent information to be wrong.

The Russian physicist Igor Suslov (1992) argued that some forms of humour – particularly puns and verbal jokes – work by drawing people into error. They are led to believe one thing, but then realise they are wrong. Humour, he argued, is a rapid emotional response that makes people aware of their initial mistake, which they then correct. Suslov's theory is consistent with some common features of humour – notably, that timing is important and hackneyed old jokes generally cease to be funny. If the timing is wrong or the joke is too familiar, people are not lured into making the initial error. The theory once again high-lights the importance of incongruity.

Humour is often associated with laughter, but the two are dis-tinctly different. Laughter is by no means synonymous with humour; indeed, it is sometimes associated with moods and situations that are far from light-hearted or humorous (Provine, 2012).

The stereotypical vocal patterns associated with human laughter emerge early in development, at 2–3 months of age. In very young children, laughter is evoked most easily by tick-ling. Robert Provine (2000) has argued that the 'ha-ha' vocal-isation of laughter has ancient biological origins, evolving from the 'pant-pant' vocalisations present in the rough-and-tumble play of chimpanzees. The 50-kHz ultrasonic vocalisations pro-duced when rats engage in rough-and-tumble play has also been regarded as a precursor of human laughter (Panksepp, 2007). This response can be evoked by tickling rats, especially in areas such as the nape of the neck. Analysis of the rats' behaviour indicates that these laughter-like high-frequency vocalisations are emitted in positive, playful social situations. In rats, these vocalisations are produced by subcortical structures (Panksepp, 2007). Robert Provine (2012) has suggested that human laughter is also generated at the subcortical level of brain organisation and that the precursors of laughter evolved a long time ago. The link between tickling and laughter has also been proposed as an important step in the evolution of humour (Gervais & Wilson, 2005).

Human laughter is primarily a social response: it is 30 times more frequent in social than in solitary situations (Provine, 2012). Laughter can be contagious – laughter causes laughter. But laughing *with* someone is very different from laughing *at* them. Laughter can be used aggressively to deride, dominate or taunt. People also laugh when they are nervous, excited or tense, and laughter can signify anxiety or submission. The quality of laughter varies and differences are readily detected in analysis of the sounds produced (Kipper & Todt, 2005). The particular sound can indicate to the listener whether the intentions of the person who is laughing are friendly or not.

Laughter, then, is a form of social communication with many different functions and it occurs in many contexts other than ones associated with humour. It follows that humour is not best judged solely by whether it produces laughter. We accept, of course, that laughter can be an expression of elevated, positive mood. It can also be a signal that what is about to come is not to be taken seriously, in a clear parallel with play signals such as the play-face in chimpanzees.

HUMOUR AS A SIGNAL

Just as friendly laughter can signal that what is about to be said is not malign, the truth can be spoken in jest when it is implicitly understood that the intent is not to wound. This ability of humour to create a sort of protected context was formalised in the practice of employing court jesters or fools in royal courts from the Egyptian Pharaohs to those of European monarchs of the Middle Ages. The jesters and fools were able to say things that others could not. As in play, the context was protected. Their licence to mock playfully meant they could humorously dispense unwelcome truths and frank good sense. They could bring bad news to the king that no one else would dare deliver. For instance, when the French fleet was destroyed by the English at the Battle of Sluys in 1340, Philippe VI's jester told him that the English sailors 'don't even have the guts to jump into the water like our brave French' (Otto, 2001). The behaviour of fools and jesters provides another parallel between humour and play. In both cases they occur in a protected context in which the behaviour is insulated from its normal consequences.

HUMOUR AND WELL-BEING

The ability to see the funny or absurd side of life relieves tension and helps people to cope with stress. The relatively few scientific studies that have delved into this area have found that humour has a range of psychological and physiological benefits, with no known harmful side-effects. Inducing enjoyment through humour can temporarily reduce stress levels and boost certain aspects of the immune system, potentially making people more resistant to infection and disease (Bennett et al., 2003; Martin, 1997).

Humour has practical benefits too. Humour in the workplace is found to be correlated with better working relationships, greater job satisfaction, increased productivity and a lower turnover of staff (Morrison, 2004). In his discussion of present-day hunter-gatherers, Peter Gray (2009) argued that they use humour, deliberately, to maintain equality and stop quarrels. Gray regarded their playfulness as crucial to maintaining social cohesion. Humour helps to build and maintain relationships, as well as making individuals more resilient. As such, it is one of factors that contribute to happiness (Martin, 2005).

HUMOUR AND PLAYFULNESS

Inasmuch as humour is original, its production is a creative act. When psychologists have analysed the relationship between creativity and humour, incongruity emerges again as a core theme (Murdock & Ganim, 1993). A clear link can be seen with playful play, where creativity is fostered by generating novel combinations of acts or ideas, accompanied by a positive mood that facilitates divergent thinking. Those who generate humour often do so playfully. To give just one example, David Jones, under his pen name of Daedulus, wrote more than 2,000 whimsical articles for *New Scientist* magazine, the *Guardian* newspaper and the journal *Nature*. His creativity, which built on his knowledge of science, was astonishing. In writing about this in his book *The Aha! Moment*, Jones (2012) frequently referred to the playfulness involved in creating the humorous scenarios.

Some evidence suggests that more creative people are better able to generate humour. In two separate studies, students were asked to supply captions to cartoons (Brodzinsky & Rubien, 1976; Treadwell, 1970). Their creativity was also assessed using Mednick's (1968) Remote Associates Test, which we described in

Chapter 5, where the task is to identify a word that connects three seemingly unrelated words. The students who performed well on this test also produced the most humorous cartoon captions. A more recent study with 86 adults similarly found a positive association between creativity and humour (Humke & Schaefer, 1996). Humour might be correlated with creativity, but can the use of humour actually *enhance* creativity? One project aimed to enhance creativity in adolescents by exposing them to humorous stories (Ziv, 1989). The adolescents did become more creative relative to a comparison group when measured on a standard test of originality. The effect was probably short-lived and may have relied on the ability of humour to elevate mood. Whether humour can have more lasting effects on creativity remains uncertain – though it is certainly plausible because humour, like play, can help people to see the world in new ways.

In their extensive review of the evolution and functions of humour, Hurley, Dennett and Adams (2011) consider its link with play. They approve of Ramachandran's (1998) theory that tickling is a form of play and that laughter evolved from being tickled. In non-human species, tickling and chasing in social play involve peaks of excitement by the tickled or the chased. The conflict between a potentially aggressive act and its non-aggressive outcome is resolved. That happy state of resolving conflicting emotions might have provided the conditions necessary for the evolution of the appreciation of humour when incongruities are resolved.

CONCLUSIONS

Like others, we doubt that a single underlying theme can explain humour, just as a single theme does not capture the entirety of play. Even so, the commonalities between playful play and the generation of humour are striking. They both encourage a positive, light-hearted mood among participants. They both occur in protected contexts where the normal consequences of the behaviour are disregarded. They are both intrinsically motivated and rewarding in their own right. And they both generate novel outcomes that can lead to creativity.

10

Dreams, drugs and creativity

Dreaming, like humour, has a number of features in common with play. It occurs in a protected context and combines existing thoughts into novel combinations, potentially providing a safe way to discover new connections and possibilities. Dreaming has been linked explicitly to creativity; many writers, artists, musicians and even some scientists have claimed that good ideas came to them in the course of dreaming (Martin, 2002). Other states of consciousness besides dreaming and wakefulness may also be occasional sources of new ideas. In this chapter we look at dreaming, daydreaming and the altered mental states induced by alcohol and other psychoactive drugs. We consider their relationship with play and their influence on creativity. Strong claims have been made by some creative people about their enhanced ability to come up with good ideas when in such states (Martin, 2008).

DREAMS

Everybody dreams but most people rapidly forget their dreams when they wake up. When dreams are remembered, they are found to consist of familiar thoughts, images and memories mixed together in unusual and sometimes bizarre ways (Martin, 2002). A person may attempt to make sense of these novel sequences and, in so doing, generate something that is genuinely creative. As Arthur Koestler (1964) described it, links are forged between disparate things that would never be connected when awake. People who would not consider themselves especially creative can be remarkably good at producing novel ideas when they dream, and some of these ideas can be harnessed in waking life. As with play, most of the novel combinations are of no practical use, but once in a while something genuinely interesting emerges. It is also worth remembering that dreaming occupies a remarkably large slice of human existence. By the time someone dies, he or she may have spent in total around 25 years asleep, of which several years will have been in the dream state (Martin, 2002).

In many of his writings, the psychologist Nicholas Humphrey (1983, 1986, 1992, 2000, 2007) has argued that dreaming brings substantial benefits in addition to those arising from memory consolidation and recovery from fatigue. His theme is that dreams often place the individual in situations that he or she has never previously encountered but might encounter at a future date. To use the term that we have applied to play behaviour, dreaming is a form of safe simulation. The experience of dreaming provides the dreamer with mental skills that might become useful later on. Humphrey explicitly drew a link between play and dreaming. He suggested that the individual is introduced to introspectively observable mental states that are as yet unfamiliar in real life. In this way, dreaming may allow imagined experiences that are beyond the scope of waking play. Developing this idea, Humphrey (2000) speculated that dreaming gives the individual the chance to discover what it is like to be the subject of strange but humanly significant mental states. In a similar vein, Revonsuo (2000) suggested that dreaming simulates threatening events, enabling the individual to discover what it is like to perceive threat and to rehearse ways of avoiding such threats.

In line with this thinking, many claims have been made that dreams have inspired creative individuals and enabled them to generate new ideas (Barrett, 2001; Martin, 2002). The surreal paintings of Salvador Dali have an explicitly dream-like quality, and Dali certainly believed that dreams inspired his work. Film-makers such as Ingmar Bergmann and Federico Fellini turned their own dream images into film sequences.

Paul McCartney heard the melody of 'Yesterday' in a dream and initially could not believe that it was a new melody rather than a memory of someone else's song. Other well-documented examples of creative solutions arising from dreams include Dmitri Mendeleyev's categorisation of chemical elements, Elias Howe's invention of the sewing machine, and Herman Hilprecht's deciphering of ancient Babylonian hieroglyphs (Van de Castle, 1994). While these accounts are anecdotal, empirical research has demonstrated a systematic relationship between dreaming and creativity.

The dreams of creative people contain a higher proportion of unusual combinations (Domino, 1976), a reminder that dreaming, like play, involves the generation of novel combinations. More generally, creativity is associated with having longer and more frequent dreams (Blagrove & Hartnell, 2000; Livingston & Levin, 1991; Schredl, 1995). Whether in such studies dreaming influenced creativity, or creativity affected dreaming, or another unknown factor influenced both, could not be determined. However, direct evidence of a link between dreaming and subsequent creativity came from a substantial retrospective study (Schredl & Erlacher, 2007). The results, derived from a specially designed questionnaire, indicated that about 8% of all remembered dreams led to subsequent creativity in waking life. The examples were of four main types:

- dream images that were used in later work
- dreams that solved a problem
- dreams that provided the impetus to do something the individual otherwise had difficulty doing
- dreams containing emotional insights.

The main factors influencing the frequency of creative dreams were the frequency of dream recall and the openness of the individual to new experiences. Such evidence supports the anecdotal accounts of many individuals that dreaming has helped them to solve problems and discover new ideas.

Creative dreaming is especially associated with the dreams that occur during the transition between wakefulness and sleep (known as hypnagogic dreams) and those occurring during the comparable transition from sleep to wakefulness (Martin, 2002). During these sleep–wake transitions, dream-like thoughts can become loosely associated, whimsical, and even bizarre. Hallucinations are common and may take the form of flashes of light or colour, sounds, voices, faces, or fully formed pictures. Mental imagery may become particularly vivid and fantastical, and a few individuals may experience synaesthesia, in which stimulation of one of the senses is experienced in another. The novel experiences and hallucinations arising during this altered state of consciousness are also more likely to be remembered and carried across into the waking state than dreams occurring in deep sleep.

Of the many examples of creativity arising from hypnagogic dreams, one of the most famous is that of August Kekulé von Stradonitz (1829–96), the discoverer of the chemical structure of the benzene ring. His theory proved to be so important that in 1890 the German Chemical Society organised a celebration in Kekulé's honour. At the celebration, Kekulé gave a speech describing how the theory came to him. He said he hit upon the ring shape of the benzene molecule after falling half asleep by the fireside and having a dream in which a snake seized its own tail (Benfey, 1958). It is possible, through attention and practice, for individuals to become more aware of the hypnagogic state as it occurs and to experience and remember their dreams more fully. The writer Robert Louis Stevenson deliberately cultivated hypnagogic dreaming in this way in order to generate new ideas for his stories; one of the best known being *The Strange Case of Dr Jekyll and Mr Hyde* (Martin, 2002).

Lucid dreaming is a particular form of dreaming in which the dreamer becomes aware at the time that they are dreaming (Hearne, 1990; LaBerge et al., 1981; Martin, 2002). The dreamer may also be able to exert some degree of control over the content of the dream (Fenwick et al., 1984). Lucid dreaming, like other forms of dreaming, is linked to creativity. The most creative student subjects in one study were significantly more likely to have lucid dreams than the less creative individuals (Blagrove & Hartnell, 2000). In his book on sleep, Martin (2002) described many examples of lucid dreaming and how this ability can be developed with practice. One particularly remarkable example was that of Hervey de Saint-Denys, a nineteenth-century French scholar who developed his lucid dreaming ability to such an extent that he could probe long-forgotten memories and conjure up all manner of pleasurable dream experiences. The memories he explored during his lucid dreams could be rearranged into new sequences that were in every sense creative. This rearrangement to form something new is analogous to what happens with play.

DAYDREAMING

Daydreaming, which occurs during waking consciousness, is a distinctly different state from dream sleep. Nonetheless, it does have certain features in common with both dreaming and play and, like them, it can facilitate creativity.

In the absence of a task that requires deliberative processing, the mind tends to wander, flitting from one thought to another with fluidity and ease – a generally pleasurable state commonly known as daydreaming. Someone who is daydreaming may be pondering on a particular theme, or their thoughts may meander randomly. Either way, their thinking is not focused on the current situation or the task in hand and, as such, it could be regarded as a waste of time. In this sense, daydreaming is analogous to play and contrasts with 'serious' problem-solving cognition. In terms of creativity, the daydream may lead the thinker further afield and enable them to stumble across new connections. When stuck on a particularly difficult problem, indulging in a good daydream isn't just an escape – it may be the most productive thing to do.

Some argue that daydreaming is a valuable tool for creativity, precisely because of its ability to make new associations and connections. Instead of focusing on the immediate surroundings, the daydreamer is free to engage in abstract thought and imaginative ramblings, picturing the future, and contemplating 'what-if' scenarios without constraints. In yet another parallel with play, the seemingly frivolous wandering of the mind could have serious benefits. One possible function of daydreaming is to plan and anticipate personally relevant future goals (Baird, Smallwood & Schooler, 2011). In line with this hypothesis, the content of daydreams is predominantly future-focused and is often useful to people later on, as they navigate through their daily lives. According to this view, daydreaming is an adaptive feature of the human mind and, like play, has potentially significant benefits that may accrue after a long delay.

Daydreaming is accompanied by a distinct pattern of brain activity. Functional magnetic resonance imaging (fMRI) shows that during daydreaming simultaneous activation occurs of regions of the brain that ordinarily are not strongly connected, facilitating communication between them. When deprived of varying sensory input, this network of different brain regions is brought together (Mason et al., 2007). The network of brain regions that become connected during daydreaming is most engaged when people are performing tasks that require little conscious attention. It has been suggested that creativity is enhanced in this state because the simultaneous activation of different brain areas enables people to understand and express novel orderly relationships (Heilman, Nadeau & Beversdorf, 2003). As in play, different ideas or ways of doing things may be brought together creatively.

CREATIVITY AND ALCOHOL

Another, distinctly different, way in which most humans experience altered states of consciousness is through their use of psychoactive drugs. In many societies, the most commonly used and publicly acceptable psychoactive drug – besides caffeine – is alcohol (Martin, 2008). Alcohol has been widely consumed in many cultures throughout human history. Wine was being made in the region of modern-day Armenia eight thousand years ago, long before the wheel was invented; and the Egyptians were drinking wine and beer six thousand years ago. Humanity's ancient and sometimes troubled relationship with alcohol revolves around its psychoactive properties. As Hugh Johnson (1989) acknowledged in his history of wine: 'It was not the subtle bouquet of wine, or a lingering aftertaste of violets and raspberries, that first caught the attention of our ancestors. It was, I'm afraid, its effect.' Humans like to consume alcohol because it makes them feel different. Moderate doses can induce a pleasant state of relaxation and reduced anxiety. Larger doses produce intoxication, with potentially dramatic mental and physical effects. Intoxication is not just about feeling good; it can be about taking a short break from sober normality (Martin, 2008).

Alcohol has featured prominently in the lives of many creative people (Beveridge & Yorston, 1999). Among the writers who famously consumed a lot were Dylan Thomas, Brendan Behan, James Joyce, Dorothy Parker, F. Scott Fitzgerald, Eugene O'Neill, Ernest Hemingway and Jack Kerouac. Visual artists who drank included Francis Bacon, Edvard Munch, Willem De Kooning, Jackson Pollock, Mark Rothko and Amedeo Modigliani. The rock musician drinkers are too numerous to mention.

Many creative people drink a lot of alcohol, but does their drinking make them more creative? Two clinicians who surveyed this field concluded that: 'If one is struck by the large number of artists who drank to excess, one is also struck by the appalling personal and physical price they paid. In fact, most artists who have experimented with creating while under the influence of alcohol have concluded that it hinders rather than aids the artistic process' (Beveridge & Yorston, 1999). On the other hand, many creative people clearly believe that alcohol has helped them to be more creative by giving them different experiences, dissociating them from everyday life and enabling them to think more deeply (Koski-Jännes, 1985). Some experimental evidence suggests that this belief has a basis in reality.

In one experimental study, which looked at a sample of scientists, mild alcohol intoxication made them significantly more creative and original in their thinking about science, affecting the incubation phase of their creativity (Norlander & Gustafson, 1998). By altering people's cognitive style, alcohol can make them temporarily less inhibited and less tied to rational and constrained ways of thinking (Gustafson &

Kallmen, 1989). Alcohol releases the shackles of conventionality. As William James (1902) observed, 'Sobriety diminishes, discriminates, and says no; drunkenness expands, unites and says yes.'[27]

The relationship between alcohol and creativity is certainly not straightforward, though. In a biographical study of 34 well-known creative people who drank heavily, the data indicated that alcohol impaired the productivity of three-quarters of the sample, especially later in life. Even so, on reflection by the people concerned, alcohol was thought to have been of direct creative benefit to 9% and indirect benefit to 50% (Ludwig, 1990). Solid evidence indicates that a small amount of alcohol can enable people to solve problems that cannot be solved by those who are sober (Jarosz, Colflesh & Wiley, 2012). In this study, the effects of moderate alcohol intoxication were tested with a creative problem-solving task. Individuals were brought to a blood alcohol content of approximately 0.75 mg of alcohol per 100 ml of blood and, after reaching peak intoxication, completed a battery of test items. Mildly intoxicated individuals solved more items, and in less time, than sober individuals. More interestingly still, they were more likely to perceive their creative solutions as the result of a sudden insight. The general conclusion from this and other studies is that moderate doses of alcohol can facilitate some aspects of creativity in some people, probably by reducing social inhibitions and enlarging the focus of attention.

OTHER DRUGS

Many other psychoactive drugs besides alcohol have been used to create altered states of consciousness in many cultures for thousands of years (Martin, 2008). Opium from the poppy, cocaine from the coca plant, mescaline from the peyote cactus, ergot from the *Claviceps* fungi that infect grasses such as rye, psilocybin from 200 species of Basidiomycota mushrooms, khat from an Arabian shrub, and many more examples all contain psychoactive chemicals.

The nineteenth century witnessed a vogue for experimenting with drugs as tools for exploring the inner workings of the mind and unleashing its creative potential (Martin, 2008). Thomas De Quincey described the pleasures and pitfalls of taking opium in *Confessions of an English Opium-Eater*. The English romantic poet, Samuel Taylor Coleridge also reported the vivid imagery of the opium experience, and the 1832 poem by Alfred Lord Tennyson, 'The lotus-eaters', describes how opium was used as a creative tool. Charles Baudelaire, who was inspired by the drug-fuelled works of Coleridge and De Quincey, relates how he and his friends used opium and hashish to help them break into unexplored realms of the human imagination and to view the world in novel ways.

The artistic tradition of using drugs to aid creativity continued in the twentieth century.[28] During the 1960s and 1970s, the creativeness of a substantial body of Western art and music was attributed to psychedelic drugs such as LSD. Some artists and musicians proclaimed themselves to be 'psychedelic artists', while others acknowledged the influence of psychedelic drug experiences on their work. In the generally more staid realm of science, LSD was used by the chemist Kary Mullis, who invented the polymerase chain reaction (PCR). This very important process, which is used in forensic investigations, amplifies small pieces of DNA by generating thousands or millions of copies of the DNA sequences. Mullis was quoted as saying: 'Would I have invented PCR if I hadn't taken LSD? I seriously doubt it' (see Mullis, 1998). Whether or not he was right (and he was wrong about many other matters such his denial of the link between HIV and AIDS), he went on to win a Nobel Prize for his work.

The influence of LSD on artistic creativity was explored in a remarkable long-term series of anecdotal case studies by the American psychiatrist Oscar Janiger. Between 1954 and 1962, Janiger organised LSD sessions for almost a thousand people between the ages of 18 and 81 years from a variety of professions including doctors, lawyers, housewives, police officers, lorry drivers, students and unemployed and retired people (Dobkin de Rios & Janiger, 2003). In contrast to the experimental approaches of many other psychedelic drug studies of this period, Janiger's took place in a naturalistic setting with the aim of exploring the nature of the 'intrinsic, characteristic LSD response'. Unsurprisingly, the volunteers' experiences varied widely, but adverse reactions were extremely rare and the vast majority described the experience as valuable and facilitating their sense of creativity. Janiger then examined the effects of LSD on creativity in a more controlled setting. He gave the drug to a mixed group of 60 visual artists. The artists' output of over 250 pictures was later analysed by a professor of art history, who compared works produced before and after the LSD sessions. The heterogeneity of the population and the value judgements inherent in analysing the art made it impossible to reach objective conclusions about how LSD affected creativity. Nonetheless, the drug did appear to enhance certain aspects of the artists' work, with a tendency towards more expressionistic work and a sharpening of colour. Particularly interesting were the many qualitative reports from the artists themselves, who, without exception, reported the LSD experience to be artistically and personally profound. We accept that they reported accurately what they felt, but an element of self-justification and willingness to please the investigators may have been involved.

In another study, 27 individuals working in professions that involved some degree of creativity were 'primed' in a pre-drug session, during which they were encouraged to select problems of professional interest that required a creative solution (Harman, McKim & Mogar, 1966). The researchers encouraged positive expectations by telling the subjects that the drug would enhance their creativity and help them to work more productively without distractions. The subjects were then given the psychedelic drug mescaline during sessions in which they were encouraged to work in groups or tackle their chosen problems individually. Within a week of the drug session, the subjects submitted a written account of their experience and, in further interviews 8 weeks later, they were asked how the drug had affected their creativity and work performance. All the participants reported that their performance had improved. In their written accounts they all described how the drug had enhanced their creative process. This study was not controlled for placebo effects and, for that reason, is difficult to evaluate. It showed how both the mind-set of the subjects and the context in which the drug is administered can affect experience.[29]

The psychological experiences of humans under the influence of psychedelic drugs are multifarious and idiosyncratic, but a broad range of common characteristics has nevertheless been identified (Sessa, 2008). These include alterations in the user's emotions, sensory perceptions in all the modalities, and perception of how different things are related. Two particular features of the psychedelic experience have special relevance to the creative process; namely, a general increase in the ability to deal with complexity, and an increase in openness such that the usual restraints that encourage humans to accept preconceived ideas are challenged. Another important feature is the tendency for users to assign unique and novel meanings to their experience (Sessa, 2008).

Evidence that psychoactive drugs can improve creativity is often equivocal. The personality of the individual, the circumstances in which they take the drug, and many other variables will influence how they are affected. Conscious expectations can have substantial effects on the subjective experience. Someone who is expecting to become more creative because of a drug may perform better than someone without such expectations, regardless of any pharmacological effects. The expectation of a positive outcome can also interact with the real effects of a drug, amplifying some of its components and diminishing others.[30]

CONCLUSIONS

This chapter has been concerned with the enhanced creativity that can flow from dreaming and other altered states of consciousness, and the analogies between these states and play. For some people, and in some contexts, altered states of consciousness do causally influence creativity. Every so often, the link with play has been explicit, but more often in the extensive research on dreaming and drugs the emphasis of investigators has been on experiences that enable people to perceive things in different ways or connect previously unrelated thoughts. Here the link with play is analogous. Dreaming and the altered states of consciousness induced by some psychoactive drugs occur in protected contexts, in the sense that novel patterns of thought can occur freely, without their conventional real-life consequences. In a dream, you can fly or walk through brick walls without hurting yourself. More importantly, thoughts may be combined in novel and sometimes fruitful ways. Research in this field has often focused on relatively short-term effects on creativity, whereas the work on animal and human play suggests that the benefits often accrue much later. Future research could usefully examine whether the creative benefits of altered states of consciousness, when they do occur, are long-lasting.[31]

11
Pulling the threads together

Our purpose has been to examine whether play, and especially playful play, enhances creativity and hence innovation. At the outset we drew a distinction between playful play, in which the mood is positive, and non-playful play in which the mood is different. We have argued that play assists creativity by generating novel combinations of thoughts or actions, or by providing experience that enables the subsequent production of novel solutions to problems.

We started with an account of the research on animal play, considering its organisation, development, function and evolution. Play is defined by pointing to examples that people readily recognise. The distinction between play and serious behaviour may be communicated between players by social signals such as the 'play-face'. Play involves novel combinations of actions or thoughts. These actions or thoughts occur outside their usual context and may be exaggerated. In social play, roles may be reversed, with the dominant individual handicapping itself. Play is typically suppressed by illness, anxiety or chronic stress and is highly sensitive to prevailing conditions. A core feature of play is its intrinsic motivation: no additional external reward is required to motivate an individual to play. Playful play is associated with a positive, light-hearted mood that facilitates divergent thinking.

Many different types of play occur in animals, as in humans. Play with objects has different characteristics from play with peers, both in its structure and when it occurs during development. The distinctiveness of different forms of play has contributed to the difficulty in defining the unifying character of play. The playful mood state may bind together different examples of playful play.

We highlighted the distinction between the motivational underpinnings of play and its biological functions. Many different explanations have been offered for the functions of play. According to one hypothesis, play enhances an individual's ability to cooperate, compete and co-exist with members of its own species, develops social skills, and cements social relationships. Another hypothesis is that play facilitates the acquisition of complex physical skills by fine-tuning neuromuscular systems and the processing of sensory information. Other potential functions include increasing the individual's knowledge of its home environment, making the individual more resistant to stress, or enlarging its behavioural repertoire and thereby making it better able to adjust to new conditions.

The particular functional hypothesis that we have explored in this book is that play provides a mechanism for generating new forms of behaviour or new ideas, enabling the individual to discover new solutions and ways of breaking out of a rut. Play, we argue, equips the individual with experiences that enable it to meet future challenges in novel ways. These and other proposed functions are not mutually exclusive, and different forms of play may bring different biological benefits during the course of an individual's lifespan. Researchers' attempts to demonstrate that any one of these proposed functions is correct have proved difficult. Nevertheless, evidence obtained from studying animals does suggest that individuals who play more are more likely to survive and reproduce.

Before leaving the biology of play, we considered how it might have evolved. Play has biological costs. A fundamental tenet of biology is that if an activity carries costs then it must have evolved because of the benefits it brings. The play activities of birds and mammals might have had a common evolutionary origin in reptilian ancestors. Alternatively, play might have evolved separately in birds and mammals and be related to the extended parental care found in both. If such care allowed the young animal to play and exercise, those that did so would be at an advantage over those that did not. A variety of benefits could have followed and driven further changes in the course of evolution. For example, testing the conditions around the young animal could have led to greater cognitive ability with more elaborately organised brains. Such behaviour could have facilitated further creativity and innovation, so driving yet more evolutionary changes in the descendants of the players. Many or all of the suggested functions of play may turn out to be real.

SOLVING DIFFICULT PROBLEMS

We described some remarkable instances of birds and non-human mammals producing creative solutions to difficult problems. Crows, parrots, dolphins, whales, monkeys and apes provide the most striking examples of individuals displaying novel and creative patterns of behaviour. All these animals are highly playful early in their lives and their early experiences may have enabled their subsequent creativity.

When it comes to humans, we argued that playful thought and playful behaviour can assist creativity and hence help individuals and organisations to be more innovative. Many of the most creative people in the arts and sciences have been highly playful and willing to break the rules of conventional behaviour. Individuals differ temperamentally, but playfulness and hence creativity can be encouraged in those who may not see themselves as being especially creative. Producing creative ideas does not necessarily lead to successful innovation, however. Innovation involves transforming creative ideas into practical outcomes that are adopted by others. Being a successful innovator requires other attributes, such as analytical skills, determination and persistence, that are different from the cognitive features underpinning creativity.

LOSS OF PLAY IN CHILDHOOD

Various commentators have expressed increasing concern that children in developed countries are being deprived of opportunities to play freely with other children outdoors. Historical changes in the play experiences of children have been driven partly by the fears of parents for the safety of their offspring and by the realities of educational pressures. Some authorities have been sceptical about the benefits of unstructured play, believing that it competes with the time needed to learn the fundamental skills of literacy and numeracy. Teaching these skills at too early an age may be a mistake. When children are ready to learn, playfulness in the classroom can have major benefits in motivating them. Breaks or recesses between lessons allow time for play and enable the children to restore their attention to what they are being taught.

Recent historical changes in childhood experiences have not been uniformly negative by any means. The potential benefits include enhanced analytical intelligence, a much greater ability to deal with technology, and the opportunity through social media to interact with larger networks of individuals. The downsides include fewer opportunities to engage in physical activity or interact in person with other children. Efforts to intervene in children's experience with the aim of increasing sociality and creativity have had mixed results, though some studies have been encouragingly positive. The evidence suggests that play does boost children's creativity, at least in the short term. Breaking rules and making new ones is a skill fostered by play and may help individuals when they are challenged later in life by circumstances they have not encountered before. Our focus has been on creativity, but children's experience of social play will have more wide-ranging effects on their ability to form successful relationships with other people later in life. Play may also affect children's motivation so that they remain interested in tasks when others who have had more limited play experience get frustrated and give up.

IMPLICATIONS FOR INDIVIDUALS AND ORGANISATIONS

The generally positive results of boosting play experiences in children have implications for adults engaged in creative activities. They suggest that the creativity of adults, like that of children, can be enhanced, at least in the short term. Encouraging playful play in groups – as distinct from 'brainstorming' and other popular techniques – can help organisations to become more creative and hence more innovative.

One way to encourage the creative process is through humour. Humour has many facets and we have not done justice to all of them in this book. Humour and play do, however, have features in common. They both involve social signals and are sensitive to prevailing conditions. Humour and playful play are both associated with a positive, light-hearted mood that facilitates divergent thinking (though it remains unclear whether the mood is exactly the same in both cases). Play and humour both occur in protected environments and are intrinsically motivated. Certain forms of humour, in common with play, rely on generating novel or incongruous combinations of thoughts. The consequences can be highly creative. These links between play, playfulness and humour may be more than mere analogies. Playfulness encourages humour and humour encourages playfulness.

Dreams can occasionally lead to creative outcomes, as can daydreaming. Many creative people have used their dreams as tools to help them discover new ideas. Dreaming, like play, occurs in a protected state and involves combining familiar memories, thoughts and ideas in novel ways. Other altered states of consciousness can be induced by psychoactive drugs such as alcohol or LSD, and strong claims have been made that they can enhance creativity. However, evidence that drug-induced altered states of consciousness do enhance creativity is often equivocal. The personality of the individual has an influence on how they are affected and the drug dose can be crucial. Conscious expectations may interact with the pharmacological effects. Despite these caveats, the evidence suggests that, for some people and in some contexts, drug-induced altered states of consciousness can causally influence creativity. After taking a drug, some individuals are able to perceive things in a different way or connect previously unrelated ideas or memories. The disinhibiting effects of some psychoactive drugs may make it easier to form associations between seemingly unrelated thoughts. Furthermore, alcohol and some other drugs can induce positive moods that assist in social interactions and creative thought. Our suggestions here are expressed with caution because they could be misinterpreted or might appear to underplay the harm caused by the abuse of alcohol and illegal drugs. Nevertheless, allowing time for daydreaming and paying attention to dreams may lead to greater productivity in the workplace, and a glass of wine may help to generate the positive mood and playfulness that we believe are important in developing new ways of thinking.

SUGGESTIONS FOR FUTURE RESEARCH

This book is about ideas drawn from many different strands of scientific research. A great deal about the biology and psychology of play, playfulness and creativity is still poorly understood. We have attempted, where possible, to base our conclusions on empirical evidence and have pointed out where evidence is lacking or incomplete. More research is undoubtedly needed before confident answers can be given to the following questions.

1. What is the role of play in the development of complex mental and physical skills? Is it the best or only way to acquire certain skills?
2. What are the optimal periods in development for different forms of play?
3. How does play differ from other forms of behaviour in terms of its motivation and control?
4. What is the nature of the positive mood associated with playful play and how does it influence creativity?
5. Do animals that play more have a better knowledge of their environment than those that play less?
6. Do individuals that play more find globally optimal solutions more easily than those that play less?
7. What is the neural basis of play and playfulness?
8. Why are some individuals generally more playful than others? Conversely, why do some individuals not play, even in suitable conditions?

9. What are the genetic and environmental influences on play and playfulness?
10. What are the genetic and environmental influences on creativity?
11. Why are some species more playful than other, closely related, species? How do these differences relate to the functions of play?
12. Are the most playful lineages of animals the ones that have evolved most rapidly?
13. What is the optimal mix of creative and innovative individuals in an organisation, society or species?
14. What are the optimal environmental conditions for creativity in humans?
15. What interventions are most effective in enhancing creativity in children, and how long-lasting are those improvements?
16. What are the links between childhood play and adult creativity?
17. How, and under what circumstances, does humour contribute to creativity?
18. How does humour relate to playfulness? Are the underlying mood states the same or similar?
19. How, and under what circumstances, does dreaming contribute to creativity? Can the contribution be enhanced?
20. How, and under what circumstances, do other altered states of consciousness, including those induced by alcohol and other psychoactive drugs, affect creativity, both in the short and long term?

Biology, psychology and the social sciences come together when exploring the links between play, playfulness, creativity and innovation. Individuals undoubtedly differ in both their playfulness and creativity, but such characteristics are not immutable. People can be helped to become more creative. However, creativity may be antithetical to the analytical intelligence required for innovation. Can people be helped to become more creative *and* more innovative? Insights from developmental psychology may provide answers, in that an individual's receptiveness to different types of training and advice change over the long period of development. Even if aptitudes for creativity and innovation are to some extent in conflict, people with different skills can complement each other in teams, as any successful organisation will show.

Facilitating playfulness through social interactions and relieving individuals of undue pressure can be important in fostering creativity. For the individual, the experiences gathered during play may not be useful immediately – although some may. Much novel behaviour and many ideas may be worthless, but some may be of great significance later on when the individual is faced with a challenge. The same ideas apply to organisations. The success of organisations relies to varying degrees on their ability to keep innovating. This ability might in future depend on how much they permit or encourage their employees to play and be playful. But, irrespective of its material benefits, the sheer fun of play provides its own satisfaction.

Notes

1. In the 1970s, two collections of psychological and sociological essays about play were published (Bruner, Jolly & Sylva, 1976; Herron & Sutton-Smith, 1971). Although some of the essays set out new ideas and results, these collections were primarily reprints of earlier articles or expressions of views that were already available. Other collections of original essays have been published more recently, notably those edited by Bornstein & O'Reilly (1993), Pellegrini (1996), Bekoff & Byers (1998)), Pellegrini & Smith (2005) and Pellegrini (2011).

2. The developmental psychologist Thomas Power (2000) in *Play and Exploration in Children and Animals* brought together animal and human literature on play. This book was important because it introduced many child psychologists to the extensive work on animals, which they had largely ignored previously. Gordon Burghardt's (2005) *The Genesis of Animal Play* defined play from his standpoint as a biologist. His definition is described in Chapter 2. With great originality he explored ideas about the evolution of play and made a case for its behavioural precursors occurring in reptiles, amphibia, fish and some invertebrates. Sergio and Vivien Pellis (2009), in *The Playful Brain*, described work on the neurobiology of play largely from studies of rats. They viewed play as the last frontier for the neurosciences. The educational psychologist, Anthony Pellegrini (2011), in *The Role of Play in Human Development*, provided an excellent review of a theoretical and empirical literature, to which he has made important contributions. He shows how opportunities for play in all its manifestations can be important for the subsequent mental and physical health of children. Finally, another major contributor to the play literature, Peter Smith (2010), offered his wise perspective on the role of play in child development in his book *Children and Play*. He adopts a middle way between the enthusiasts for play and those who are sceptical about its benefits.

3. Burghardt's criteria are as follows:

    1. The performance of the behaviour is not fully functional in the form or context in which it is expressed; that is, it includes elements, or is directed toward stimuli, that do not contribute to current survival.
    2. The behaviour is spontaneous, voluntary, intentional, pleasurable, rewarding and done for its own sake.

3. The behaviour differs from the 'serious' behaviour typical of the animal's species structurally or temporally in at least one respect: it is incomplete, exaggerated, awkward, or precocious; or it involves behaviour patterns with modified form, sequencing or targeting.

4. The behaviour is performed repeatedly in a similar but not rigidly stereotyped form during at least a portion of the animal's development.

5. The behaviour is initiated when an animal is adequately fed, healthy and free from stress. The animal is in a relaxed state.

4. Examples of playful interactions between different species can easily be found on YouTube. For instance, search for 'Deer and dog playing'.

5. John Fentress has described play in adult wolves (personal communication), Marc Bekoff in coyotes (personal communication), and one of us has observed play in adult Cape hunting dogs.

6. Burghardt (2005) has written interestingly about these motivational issues and has highlighted areas where new research is needed.

7. In his book, Power (2000) did not distinguish between questions about biological function and questions about evolution. Burghardt (2005) did, and our discussions complement what he wrote.

8. A number of other examples of animal innovation were collected in an attractive book edited by Simon Reader and Kevin Laland (2003a).

9. The logic has been examined in computer simulations. The models of Robert Fagen (1981) involved a single genetic locus with two alternative forms, or alleles, determining the presence or absence of the ability to invent through play new behavioural acts or skills. In one model, no cultural dissemination of the innovative act occurred. In a second model, invented behaviour patterns were transmitted transgenerationally from parent to offspring and intragenerationally from performer to peer. The frequency of the 'play' allele variant increased when the variant was rare. As the discovery spread in the population, playful animals lost their relative advantage because they retained the cost of playing but no longer enjoyed sole possession of the benefits because others could copy them. The frequency of the 'play' allele continued to drop until a new type of discovery was made. Fagen concluded that a play allele would become frequent only if discoveries were frequent, most discoveries were significantly beneficial, and copying by others was sufficiently selective or delayed that benefits would not accrue too rapidly to unrelated, non-playing members of the species. Like all such models, the conclusion depends on the starting assumptions. If play evolved for other reasons, such as practising complex adult behaviour, then the conditions for the evolution of play through its impact on creativity would be less stringent. Furthermore, some individuals might be able to generate creative solutions at greater speed and lower cost than others, with the consequence that they would have a differential advantage in terms of survival and reproductive success.

10. Correlational analyses could use the various play and life-history features of individual species as data points, correcting for the statistical interdependence among closely related species. The link between inventiveness and relative brain size in birds and primates described earlier in the chapter suggests that such an approach would be profitable.

11. Burghardt and his colleagues plan an expanding publicly available database that will include information on habitat, social organisation, diet, body size and brain metrics as well as the incidence of different types of play.

12. Spalding's article is also historically important because it provided the first clear account of behavioural imprinting with which Konrad Lorenz (1935) is typically associated.

13. Baldwin (1902) continued to develop his thinking and the conjecture became known as the Baldwin effect. Given Spalding's (1873) precedence and the simultaneous appearance in 1896 of Baldwin's ideas about 'organic selection', it seems inappropriate to term the evolutionary process the Baldwin effect. The trouble is that calling the proposed process the Spalding effect (or the Baldwin effect) is not descriptive of what initiates the hypothetical evolutionary process. It therefore seems more appropriate to employ a term that captures the adaptability of the organism in the evolutionary process and, to this end, the term 'adaptability driver' is used in this book.

14. A meta-analysis combines the results from a large number of published studies. Such studies can suffer from bias, since negative findings are not usually published. Nevertheless, they are generally regarded as providing a good overview of a given field when no cherry-picking of the studies driven by a particular agenda is suspected.

15. Poets and visual artists did not share the same inability to experience pleasure or lack of drive that characterised the psychiatric patients. This difference might have been due to the drugs taken by the patients.

16. The genes coded for catechol-O-methyltransferase, tryptophan hydroxylase, dopamine transporter and dopamine receptor.

17. With its buccal cavity full, the whale closes its mouth and forces all the water out by straining it through the baleen that hangs from the palate. This keeps all the food inside while getting rid of the water. At this point, the whales can swallow their food.

18. In most of the animal literature concerned with the emergence of novel patterns of behaviour, no distinction is drawn between creativity and innovation. Indeed, creativity is rarely mentioned. Reader and Laland (2003b) defined innovation as a process that results in new or modified learned behaviour and introduces novel behavioural variants into a population's repertoire. In seeking to refine this definition Ramsey, Bastian and van Schaik (2007) distinguished process and product. The 'processes' on which they focused occurred in individuals and were different from those mechanisms involved in social learning and environmental induction. We think that Ramsey et al.'s 'process' is similar to what we call creativity. They quote the evidence that of 606 cases of individual innovation in non-human primates, only 16% had spread to at least one other individual (Laland & Hoppitt, 2003; Reader & Laland, 2002). Even if the creative acts of some individuals were implemented for those individuals' own purposes, in the majority of cases they were not implemented by others. Implementation by other individuals would be Ramsey et al.'s 'product' and captured by Reader and Laland's definition of innovation. We accept that measuring creativity as distinct from innovation is difficult in animals, since the initial stage involving the performance of a creative act is usually not seen. The exceptions are the novel bubble-blowing behaviour patterns expressed by dolphins, the introduction of new syllables into birdsong, and the addition of novel items into the bowers of male bowerbirds.

19. The birth order effect was not true for girls, but girls were likely to be more playful if their mothers were younger.

20. Another group process used by many organisations for generating ideas or valuable material is 'crowd sourcing'. An organisation proposes a task to a heterogeneous group of individuals of varying knowledge and number, often via the internet (although an early example was material generated for the Oxford English Dictionary). Responding is voluntary. Those who respond may sometimes be paid but they often participate for intrinsic rewards or for social recognition. The organisation that initiates the process aims to benefit from the quality of the material that is generated.

21. Much of this research is summarised in Fagerberg, Mowery and Nelson (2005).

22. The role of play in education has engaged numerous writers from a variety of backgrounds over many years. Two prominent developmental psychologists wrote powerfully about the importance of play. Lev Vygotsky (1967) believed that literacy and imagination derived from the actions involved in play. Jean Piaget also argued that play was important in the development of the child's imagination (Piaget, 1962). In recent years, the literature has expanded rapidly and thinking has been greatly helped by the publication of two important books (Pellegrini, 2009; Smith, 2010) and by huge improvements in methodology (Lillard et al., 2012).

23. Each playful child was matched with a less playful child who was of the same intelligence, sex, age and race and had the same teacher.

24. The effects of the intervention in Garaigordobil's work were similar in boys and girls, despite big differences in the way that boys and girls play, as found in numerous studies (see Pellegrini, 2009; Power, 2000). As always in such research, a distinction must be drawn between structured play activities in the school environment and free play away from school, where the benefits might be quite different.

25. In commenting on this study, one reader of our draft manuscript believed that the children were not playing during the interventions. Another felt that the children were merely being trained for tests given at the end of the year-long intervention. Although their criticisms may have some substance, we feel that some of the games given to the children involved considerable playfulness on their part and some of the tests, such as painting, involved considerable creativity.

26. This joke and others can be found at <www.laughlab.co.uk>. Many other jokes are quoted by Hurley, Dennett and Adams (2011).

27. We suspect that William James meant by 'drunkenness' mildly intoxicated, not stupifyingly drunk.

28. The French poet and playwright Antonin Artaud made extensive use of opium and peyote, which contains the psychedelic drug mescaline (Artaud, 1976). Aldous Huxley used his own experiences with mescaline when writing *The Doors of Perception* (1954) and its sequel *Heaven and Hell* (1956).

29. Sessa (2008) argued that studies that deliberately or unintentionally disregard these factors and report negative outcomes ought not to be used as evidence to dispute the positive potential of psychedelic drugs. In general the research raised important issues to do with the way in which such studies are designed, such as selection of the subjects and investigating the interaction between their mind-set and the experiences which they are about to receive.

30. The interaction between expectation and intake of a substance means that the conventional double-blind experimental design, in which both

experimenter and subject are unaware of whether the drug or a placebo has been administered, can produce misleading results.

31. Given the potential for misunderstanding, it is perhaps necessary for us to confirm that we are not advocating the excessive consumption of alcohol or the use of illegal drugs to boost creativity.

References

Alves, J., Marques, M. J., Saur, I. & Marques, P. (2007). Creativity and innovation through multidisciplinary and multisectoral cooperation. *Creativity and Innovation Management*, 16, 27–34.

Amabile, T., Conti, R., Coon, H., Lazenby, J. & Herron, M. (1996). Assessing the work environment for creativity. *Academy of Management Journal*, 39, 1154–84.

Amundson, R. (2005). *The changing role of the embryo in evolutionary thought: roots of Evo-Devo*. Cambridge: Cambridge University Press.

Anning, A. (2010). Play and legislated curriculum. In J. Moyles (Ed.), *The excellence of play*. 3rd edition (pp. 19–33). Maidenhead, UK: Open University Press.

Artaud, A. (1976). *The peyote dance*. New York: Farrar, Straus and Giroux.

Auersperg, A. M. I., von Bayern, A. M. P., Gajdon, G. K., Huber, L. & Kacelnik, A. (2011). Flexibility in problem solving and tool use of kea and New Caledonian crows in a multi-access box paradigm. *PLoS ONE*, 6, e20231.

Auger, A. P. & Olesen, K. M. (2009). Brain sex differences and the organisation of juvenile social play behaviour. *Journal of Neuroendocrinology*, 21, 519–25.

Avital, E. & Jablonka, E. (2000). *Animal traditions: behavioural inheritance in evolution*. Cambridge: Cambridge University Press.

Baas, M., De Dreu, C. K. W. & Nijstad, B. A. (2008). A meta-analysis of 25 years of mood–creativity research: hedonic tone, activation, or regulatory focus? *Psychological Bulletin*, 134, 779–806.

Baird, B., Smallwood, J. & Schooler, J. W. (2011). Back to the future: autobiographical planning and the functionality of mind-wandering. *Consciousness & Cognition*, 20, 1604–11.

Baldwin, J. D. & Baldwin, J. I. (1977). The role of learning phenomena in the ontogeny of exploration and play. In S. Chevalier-Skolnikoff & F. E. Poirier (Eds.), *Primate bio-social development* (pp. 343–406). New York: Garland.

Baldwin, J. M. (1896). A new factor in evolution. *American Naturalist*, 30, 441–51, 536–53.

Baldwin, J. M. (1902). *Development and evolution*. London: Macmillan.

Barnett, L. A. & Kleiber, D. A. (1984). Playfulness and the early play environment. *Journal of Genetic Psychology*, 144, 153–64.

Barrett, D. (2001). *The committee of sleep: how artists, scientists, and athletes use dreams for creative problem-solving – and how you can too*. New York: Crown.

Barrett, L., Dunbar, R. M. & Dunbar, P. (1992). Environmental influences on play behaviour in immature gelada baboons. *Animal Behaviour*, 44, 111–15.

Barrett, P. & Bateson, P. (1978). The development of play in cats. *Behaviour*, 66, 106–20.

Bartholomew, G. (1982). Scientific innovation and creativity: a zoologist's point of view. *American Zoologist*, 22, 227–35.

Bateson, P. (1981). Discontinuities in development and changes in the organization of play in cats. In K. Immelmann, G. W. Barlow, L. Petrinovich & M. Main (Eds.), *Behavioral development* (pp. 281–95). Cambridge: Cambridge University Press.

Bateson, P. (2000a). Behavioural development in the cat. In D. C. Turner & P. Bateson (Eds.), *The domestic cat: the biology of its behaviour*. 2nd edition (pp. 10–22). Cambridge: Cambridge University Press.

Bateson, P. (2000b). What must be known in order to understand imprinting? In C. Heyes & L. Huber (Eds.), *The evolution of cognition* (pp. 85–102). Cambridge, MA: MIT Press.

Bateson, P. (2004). The active role of behaviour in evolution. *Biology and Philosophy*, 19, 283–98.

Bateson, P. (2006). The adaptability driver: links between behaviour and evolution. *Biological Theory: Integrating Development, Evolution and Cognition*, 1, 342–5.

Bateson, P. (2011). Theories of play. In A. D. Pellegrini (Ed.), *The Oxford handbook of the development of play* (pp. 41–47). New York: Oxford University Press.

Bateson, P., Barker, D., Clutton-Brock, T., Deb, D., D'Udine, B., Foley, R. A., et al. (2004). Developmental plasticity and human health. *Nature*, 430, 419–21.

Bateson, P. & Gluckman, P. (2011). *Plasticity, robustness, development and evolution*. Cambridge: Cambridge University Press.

Bateson, P. & Martin, P. (1999). *Design for a life: how behaviour develops*. London: Jonathan Cape.

Bateson, P., Martin, P. & Young, M. (1981). Effects of interrupting cat mothers' lactation with bromocriptine on the subsequent play of their kittens. *Physiology and Behavior*, 27, 841–5.

Bateson, P., Mendl, M. & Feaver, J. (1990). Play in the domestic cat is enhanced by rationing the mother during lactation. *Animal Behaviour*, 40, 514–25.

Bateson, P. & Young, M. (1981). Separation from mother and the development of play in cats. *Animal Behaviour*, 29, 173–80.

Batey, M. & Furnham, A. (2006). Creativity, intelligence, and personality: a critical review of the scattered literature. *Genetic, Social, and General Psychology Monographs*, 132, 355–429.

Batey, M. & Furnham, A. (2008). The relationship between measures of creativity and schizotypy. *Personality and Individual Differences*, 45, 816–21.

Bauer, E. B. & Smuts, B. K. (2007). Cooperation and competition during dyadic play in domestic dogs, *Canis familiaris*. *Animal Behaviour*, 73, 489–99.

Bekoff, M. (1976). Animal play: problems and perspectives. *Perspectives in Ethology*, 2, 165–88.

Bekoff, M. (2010). *The animal manifesto: six reasons for expanding our compassion footprint*. Novato, CA: New World Library.

Bekoff, M. & Byers, J. A. (1998). *Animal play: evolutionary, comparative, and ecological perspectives*. Cambridge: Cambridge University Press.

Bell, H. C., McCaffrey, D. R., Forgie, M. L., Kolb, B. & Pellis, S. M. (2009). The role of the medial prefrontal cortex in the play fighting of rats. *Behavioral Neuroscience*, 123, 1158–68.

Bell, H. C., Pellis, S. M. & Kolb, B. (2010). Juvenile peer play experience and the development of the orbitofrontal and medial prefrontal cortices. *Behavioural Brain Research*, 207, 7–13.

Belton, T. (2001). Television and imagination: an investigation of the medium's influence on children's story-making. *Media Culture & Society*, 23, 799–820.

Benfey, O. T. (1958). August Kekulé and the birth of the structural theory of organic chemistry in 1858. *Journal of Chemical Education*, 35, 21-3.

Bennett, M. P., Zeller, J. M., Rosenberg, L. & McCann, J. (2003). The effect of mirthful laughter on stress and natural killer cell activity. *Alternative Therapies, Health & Medicine*, 9, 38–45.

Bergen, D. (2009). Play as the learning medium for future scientists, mathematicians and engineers. *American Journal of Play*, 1, 413–28.

Beveridge, A. & Yorston, G. (1999). I drink, therefore I am: alcohol and creativity. *Journal of the Royal Society of Medicine*, 92, 646–8.

Birch, H. G. (1945). The relation of previous experience to insightful problem-solving. *Journal of Comparative Psychology*, 38, 367–83.

Bird, C. D. & Emery, N. J. (2009). Rooks use stones to raise the water level to reach a floating worm. *Current Biology*, 19, 1410–14.

Blagrove, M. & Hartnell, S. J. (2000). Lucid dreaming: associations with internal locus of control, need for cognition and creativity. *Personality & Individual Differences*, 28, 41-7.

Blatchford, P. & Baines, E. (2006). *A follow up national survey of breaktimes in primary and secondary schools*. London: The Nuffield Foundation.

Bornstein, M. H. & O'Reilly, A. W. (1993). *The role of play in the development of thought*. San Francisco, CA: Jossey-Bass.

Brodzinsky, D. M. & Rubien, J. (1976). Humor production as a function of sex of subject, creativity, and cartoon content. *Journal of Consulting and Clinical Psychology*, 44, 597–600.

Bronson, P. & Merryman, A. (2010). The creativity crisis. *Newsweek*, 10 July 2010.

Brown, S. (2009). *Play*. London: Penguin.

Brownlee, A. (1954). Play in domestic cattle: an analysis of its nature. *British Veterinary Journal*, 110, 48–68.

Bruner, J. S., Jolly, A. & Sylva, K. (1976). *Play: its role in development and evolution*. Harmondsworth, UK: Penguin.

Burdette, H. L. & Whitaker, R. C. (2005). Resurrecting free play in young children. *Archives of Pediatric and Adolescent Medicine*, 159, 46–50.

Burghardt, G. M. (2005). *The genesis of animal play: testing the limits*. Cambridge, MA: MIT Press.

Burghardt, G. M. (in press). The origins, evolution, and interconnections of play and ritual: setting the stage. In C. Renfrew, M. Boyd & I. Morley (Eds.), *Play, ritual and belief, in animals and early human societies* (pp. 000–000). Cambridge: Cambridge University Press.

Bus, R. R., Sun, W. & Oppenheim, R. W. (2006). Adaptive roles of programmed cell death during nervous system development. *Annual Review of Neuroscience*, 29, 1–35.

Busch, H. & Silver, B. (1994). *Why cats paint: a theory of feline aesthetics*. London: Weidenfeld & Nicolson.

Cameron, E. Z., Linklater, W. L., Stafford, K. J. & Minot, E. O. (2008). Maternal investment results in better foal condition through increased play behaviour in horses. *Animal Behaviour*, 76, 1511–18.

Campbell, D. T. (1960). Blind variation and selective retention in creative thought as in other knowledge processes. *Psychological Review*, 67, 380–400.

Caro, T. M. (1980). Predatory behaviour in domestic cat mothers. *Behaviour*, 74, 128–48.

Caro, T. M. (1995). Short-term costs and correlates of play in cheetahs. *Animal Behaviour*, 49, 333–45.

Caro, T. M. & Bateson, P. (1986). Organisation and ontogeny of alternative tactics. *Animal Behaviour*, 34, 1483–99.

Caro, T. M., Roper, R., Young, M. & Dank, G. R. (1979). Inter-observer reliability. *Behaviour*, 69, 303–15.

Carson, S. H., Peterson, J. B. & Higgins, D. M. (2003). Decreased latent inhibition is associated with increased creative achievement in high-functioning individuals. *Journal of Personality and Social Psychology*, 85, 499–506.

Chalmers, N. R. (1980). The ontogeny of play in feral olive baboons (*Papio anubis*). *Animal Behaviour*, 28, 570–85.

Cheke, L. D., Bird, C. D. & Clayton, N. S. (2011). Tool-use and instrumental learning in the Eurasian jay (*Garrulus glandarius*). *Animal Cognition*, 14, 441–55.

Clements, R. (2004). An investigation of the status of outdoor play. *Contemporary Issues in Early Childhood*, 5, 68–80.

Colby, R. S. & Colby, R. (2008). A pedagogy of play: integrating computer games into the writing classroom. *Computers and Composition*, 25, 300–12.

Copeland, K. A. Sherman, S. N., Kendeigh, C. K., Kalkwarf, H. J. & Saelens, B. E. (2012). Societal values and policies may curtail preschool children's physical activity in child care centers. *Pediatrics*, 129, 265–74.

Csikszentmihalyi, M. (1996). *Creativity: flow and the psychology of discovery and invention*. New York: HarperCollins.

Darwin, C. (1877). A biographical sketch of an infant. *Mind*, 2, 285–94.

Davis, M. A. (2009). Understanding the relationship between mood and creativity. *Organizational Behavior and Human Decision Processes*, 108, 25–38.

de Oliveira, C. R., Ruiz-Miranda, C. R., Kleiman, D. G. & Beck, B. B. (2003). Play behavior in juvenile golden lion tamarins (Callitrichidae: Primates): organization in relation to costs. *Ethology*, 109, 593–612.

Deag, J. M., Lawrence, C. E. & Manning, A. (1987). The consequences of differences in litter size for the nursing cat and her kittens. *Journal of Zoology*, 213, 153–79.

Deci, E. L., Koestner, R. & Ryan, R. M. (1999). A meta-analytic review of experiments examining the effects of extrinsic rewards on intrinsic motivation. *Psychological Bulletin*, 125, 627–68.

Diamond, J. & Bond, A. B. (2003). A comparative analysis of social play in birds. *Behaviour*, 140, 899–924.

Diehl, M. & Stroebe, W. (1991). Productivity loss in idea-generating groups: tracking down the blocking effect. *Journal of Personality and Social Psychology*, 61, 392–403.

Dobkin de Rios, M. & Janiger, O. (2003). *LSD, spirituality and the creative process*. Rochester, VT: Park Street Press.

Domino, G. (1976). Primary process thinking in dream reports as related to creative achievement. *Journal of Consulting and Clinical Psychology*, 44, 929–32.

Dudink, S., Simonse, H., Marks, I., de Jonge, F. H. & Spruijt, B. M. (2006). Announcing the arrival of enrichment increases play behaviour and reduces weaning-stress-induced behaviours of piglets directly after weaning. *Applied Animal Behaviour Sciences*, 101, 86–101.

Egan, J. (1976). Object-play in cats. In J. S. Bruner, A. Jolly & K. Sylva (Eds.), *Play: its role in development and evolution* (pp. 161–5). Harmondsworth, UK: Penguin.

Einon, D. & Morgan, M. (1976). Habituation of object contact in socially-reared and isolated rats (*Rattus norvegicus*). *Animal Behaviour*, 24, 415–20.

Einon, D. & Potegal, M. (1991). Enhanced defense in adult-rats deprived of play-fighting experience as juveniles. *Aggressive Behavior*, 17, 27–40.

Elkind, D. (2008). *The power of play: how spontaneous, imaginative activities lead to happier, healthier children*. Cambridge, MA: De Capo Lifelong.

Epstein, R., Kirshnit, C. E., Lanza, R. P. & Rubin, L. C. (1984). 'Insight' in the pigeon: antecedents and determinants of an intelligent performance. *Nature*, 308, 61–2.

Erikson, E. H. (1963). *Childhood and society*. New York: Norton.

Escher, M. C. (1989). *Escher on Escher: exploring the infinite*. New York: Abrams.

Eysenck, H. J. (1995). *Genius: the natural history of creativity*. Cambridge: Cambridge University Press.

Fagen, R. (1981). *Animal play behavior*. New York: Oxford University Press.

Fagen, R. & Fagen, J. (2004). Juvenile survival and benefits of play behaviour in brown bears, *Ursus arctos. Evolutionary Ecology Research*, 6, 89–102.

Fagen, R. & Fagen, J. (2009). Play behaviour and multi-year juvenile survival in free-ranging brown bears, *Ursus arctos. Evolutionary Ecology Research*, 11, 1–15.

Fagen, R. M. (1974). Selective and evolutionary aspects of animal play. *American Naturalist*, 108, 850–8.

Fagerberg, J. (2005). Innovation: a guide to the literature. In J. Fagerberg, D. C. Mowery & R. R. Nelson (Eds.), *The Oxford handbook of innovation*. Oxford: Oxford University Press.

Fagerberg, J., Mowery, D. C. & Nelson, R. R. (2005). *The Oxford handbook of innovation*. Oxford: Oxford University Press.

Fedigan, L. (1972). Social and solitary play in a colony of vervet monkeys (*Cercopithecus aethiops*). *Primates*, 13, 347–64.

Feist, G. J. (1998). A meta-analysis of personality in scientific and artistic creativity. *Personality and Social Psychology Review*, 2, 290–309.

Fenwick, P. B. C., Schatzman, M., Worsley, A., Adams, J., Stone, S. & Baker, A. (1984). Lucid dreaming: correspondence between dreamed and actual events in one subject during REM sleep. *Biological Psychology*, 18, 243–52.

Fernald, R. D. (2000). Evolution of eyes. *Current Opinion in Neurobiology*, 10, 444–50.

Fertl, D. & Wilson, B. (1997). Bubble use during prey capture by a lone bottlenose dolphin (*Tursiops truncatus*). *Aquatic Mammals*, 23, 113–14.

Feynman, R. (1985). *Surely you're joking, Mr. Feynman!* New York: Norton.

Fisher, E. P. (1992). The impact of play on development: a metaanalysis. *Play & Culture*, 5, 159–81.

Flynn, J. R. (1987). Massive IQ gains in 14 nations: what IQ tests really measure. *Psychological Bulletin*, 101, 171–91.

Forabosco, G. (1992). Cognitive aspects of the humor process: the concept of incongruity. *Humor*, 5, 45–68.

Frith, C. B. & Frith, D. W. (2004). *Bowerbirds*. Oxford: Oxford University Press.

Furedi, F. (2001). *Paranoid parenting*. London: Penguin.

Furnham, F. & Bachtiar, V. (2008). Personality and intelligence as predictors of creativity. *Personality and Individual Differences*, 45, 613–17.

Garaigordobil, M. (2006). Intervention in creativity with children aged 10 and 11 years: impact of a play program on verbal and graphic–figural creativity. *Creativity Research Journal*, 18, 329–45.

Geist, V. (1978). On weapons, combat, and ecology. In L. Krames, P. Pliner & T. Alloway (Eds.), *Aggression, dominance and individual spacing* (pp. 1–30). New York: Plenum.

George, J. M. & Zhou, J. (2002). Understanding when bad moods foster creativity and good ones don't: the role of context and clarity of feelings. *Journal of Applied Psychology*, 87, 687–97.

Gervais, M. & Wilson, D. S. (2005). The evolution and functions of laughter and humor: a synthetic approach. *Quarterly Review of Biology*, 80, 395–430.

Gilbert, S. F. (2005). Mechanisms for the environmental regulation of gene expression: ecological aspects of animal development. *Journal of Biosciences*, 30, 65–74.

Gleave, J. (2009). *Children's time to play: a literature review*. London: Play England.

Gluckman, P. & Hanson, M. (2006). *Mismatch: why our world no longer fits our bodies*. Oxford: Oxford University Press.

Gomendio, M. (1988). The development of different types of play in gazelles: implications for the nature and functions of play. *Animal Behaviour*, 36, 825–36.

Gomendio, M., Cassinello, J., Smith, M. W. & Bateson, P. (1995). Maternal state affects intestinal changes of rat pups at weaning. *Behavioral Ecology and Sociobiology*, 37, 71–80.

Graves, P. L. (1976). Nutrition, infant behavior, and maternal characteristics: a pilot study in West Bengal, India. *American Journal of Clinical Nutrition*, 29, 305–19.

Gray, P. (2009). Play as a foundation for hunter-gatherer social existence. *American Journal of Play*, 1, 476–522.

Gray, P. (2011). The decline of play and the rise of psychopathology in children and adolescents. *American Journal of Play*, 3, 443–63.

Green, R. E., Krause, J., Briggs, A. W., Maricic, T., Stenzel, U., Kircher, M., et al. (2010). A draft sequence of the Neandertal genome. *Science*, 328, 710–22.

Groos, K. (1898). *The play of animals*. New York: Appleton.

Guilford, J. P. (1956). Structure of intellect. *Psychological Bulletin*, 53, 267–93.

Gustafson, R. & Kallmen, H. (1989). The effect of alcohol intoxication on primary and secondary processes in male social drinkers. *British Journal of Addiction*, 84, 1507–13.

Harcourt, R. (1991a). The development of play in the South American fur seal. *Ethology*, 88, 191–202.

Harcourt, R. (1991b). Survivorship costs of play in the South American fur seal. *Animal Behaviour*, 42, 509–11.

Hargadon, A. & Sutton, R. I. (2000). Building an innovation factory. *Harvard Business Review*, 78, 157–66.

Harman, W. W., McKim, R. H. & Mogar, R. E. (1966). Psychedelic agents in creative problem-solving: a pilot study. *Psychological Reports*, 19, 211–27.

Hart, B. L. & Miller, M. F. (1985). Behavioral profiles of dog breeds. *Journal of the Veterinary Medicine Association*, 186, 1175–80.

Hausberger, M., Fureix, C., Bourjade, M., Wessel-Robert, S. & Richard-Yris, M.-A. (2012). On the significance of adult play: what does social play tell us about adult horse welfare? *Naturwissenschaften*, 99, 291–302.

Hearne, K. M. T. (1990). *The dream machine*. Wellingborough, UK: Aquarian Press.

Heilman, K. M., Nadeau, S. E. & Beversdorf, D. O. (2003). Creative innovation: possible brain mechanisms. *Neurocase*, 9, 369–79.

Held, S. D. E., & Spinka, M. (2011). Animal play and animal welfare. *Animal Behaviour*, 81, 891–99.

Henig, R. M. (2008). Taking play seriously. *New York Times Magazine*, February 27, 2008.

Herron, R. E. & Sutton-Smith, B. E. (1971). *Child's play*. New York: Wiley.

Hinde, R. A. & Fisher, J. (1951). Further observations on the opening of milk bottles by birds. *British Birds*, 44, 393–6.

Hinton, G. E. & Nowlan, S. J. (1987). How learning can guide evolution. *Complex Systems* 1, 495–502.

Holzhaider, J. C., Hunt, G. R. & Gray, R. D. (2010). The development of pandanus tool manufacture in wild New Caledonian crows. *Behaviour*, 147, 553–86.

Hoof, J. A. R. A. M. (1973). A structural analysis of the social behaviour of a semi-captive group of chimpanzees. In M. von Cranach & I. Vine (Eds.), *Social communication and movement: studies of interaction and expression in man and chimpanzee* (pp. 75–162). London: Academic Press.

Huber, L., Rechberger, S. & Taborsky, M. (2001). Social learning affects object exploration and manipulation in keas, *Nestor notabilis*. *Animal Behaviour*, 62, 945–54.

Huizinga, J. (1955). *Homo ludens*. Boston, MA: Beacon Press.

Humke, C. & Schaefer, C. E. (1996). Sense of humor and creativity. *Perceptual and Motor Skills*, 82, 544–6.

Humphrey, N. (1983). *Consciousness regained: chapters in the development of mind*. Oxford: Oxford University Press.

Humphrey, N. (1986). *The inner eye*. London: Faber & Faber.

Humphrey, N. (1992). *A history of the mind*. London: Chatto & Windus.

Humphrey, N. (2000). Dreaming as play. *Behavioral & Brain Sciences*, 23, 953.

Humphrey, N. (2007). Dreaming to learn. In L. Margulis & E. Punset (Eds.), *Mind, life and universe: conversations with great scientists of our time* (pp. 140–8). White River Junction, VT: Chelsea Green Publishing.

Humphreys, A. P. & Einon, D. F. (1981). Play as a reinforcer for maze-learning in juvenile rats. *Animal Behaviour*, 29, 259–70.

Hunt, G. R. (1996). Manufacture and use of hook-tools by New Caledonian crows. *Nature* 379, 249–51.

Hurley, M. M., Dennett, D. C. & Adams, R. B. (2011). *Inside jokes: using humor to reverse-engineer the mind*. Cambridge, MA: MIT Press.

Isen, A. M. & Reeve, J. (2005). The influence of positive affect on intrinsic and extrinsic motivation: facilitating enjoyment of play, responsible work behavior, and self-control. *Motivation and Emotion*, 29, 297–325.

Jablonka, E. & Raz, G. (2009). Transgenerational epigenetic inheritance: prevalence, mechanisms, and implications for the study of heredity and evolution. *Quarterly Review of Biology*, 84, 131–76.

James, W. (1902). *The varieties of religious experience*. London: Longmans, Green.

Jarosz, A. F., Colflesh, G. J. H. & Wiley, J. (2012). Uncorking the muse: alcohol intoxication facilitates creative problem solving. *Consciousness and Cognition*, 31, 487–93.

Jensen, M. B. (1999). Effects of confinement on rebounds of locomotor behaviour of calves and heifers, and the spatial preferences of calves. *Applied Animal Behaviour Science*, 62, 43–56.

Johnson, H. (1989). *The story of wine*. London: Mitchell Beazley.

Johnson, S. (2010). *Where good ideas come from*. London: Penguin.

Jones, D. (2012). *The aha! moment: a scientist's take on creativity*. Baltimore, MD: Johns Hopkins University Press.

Judson, H. F. (1980). *The search for solutions*. New York: Holt, Rinehart & Winston.

Kahlenberg, S. M. & Wrangham, R. W. (2010). Sex differences in chimpanzees' use of sticks as play objects resemble those of children. *Current Biology*, 20, R1067–R1068.

Kahneman, D. (2011). *Thinking, fast and slow*. London: Allen Lane.

Kangas, M. (2010). Creative and playful learning: learning through game co-creation and games in a playful learning environment. *Thinking Skills and Creativity*, 5, 1–15.

Kanter, R. M. (2006). Innovation: the classic traps. *Harvard Business Review*, 84, 73–83.

Kanter, R. M. (2009). *SuperCorp*. London: Profile.

Kauffman, S. A. (2000). *Investigations*. New York: Oxford University Press.

Kawecki, T. J. (2010). Evolutionary ecology of learning: insights from fruit flies. *Population Ecology*, 52, 15–25.

Kelley, T. (2006). *The ten faces of innovation: IDEO's strategies for beating the Devil's advocate & driving creativity throughout your organization*. London: Profile Books.

Kendall, R. L., Coe, R. L. & Laland, K. N. (2005). Age differences in neophilia, exploration, and innovation in family groups of callitrichid monkeys. *American Journal of Primatology*, 66, 167–88.

Kenward, B., Rutz, C., Weir, A. A. S. & Kacelnik, A. (2006). Development of tool use in New Caledonian crows: inherited action patterns and social influences. *Animal Behaviour*, 72, 1329–43.

Kim, K. H. (2005). Learning from each other: creativity in East Asian and American education. *Creativity Research Journal*, 17, 337–47.

Kim, K. H. (2011). The creativity crisis: the decrease in creative thinking scores on the Torrance tests of creative thinking. *Creativity Research Journal*, 23, 285–95.

King, Z. (2012). The Goldilocks network. *New Scientist*, 26 May 2012, 37–9.

Kipper, S. & Todt, D. (2005). The sound of laughter: recent concepts and findings in research into laughter vocalizations. In T. Garfitt, E. McMorran & J. Taylor (Eds.), *The anatomy of laughter* (pp. 24–33). London: Legenda, Modern Humanities Research Association and Maney Publishing.

Koestler, A. (1964). *The act of creation*. London: Hutchison.

Köhler, W. (1925). *The mentality of apes*. London: Paul, Trench & Trubner.

Koski-Jännes, A. (1985). Alcohol and literary creativity: the Finnish experience. *Journal of Creative Behavior*, 19, 120–36.

Kuczaj, S. A., Makecha, R., Trone, M., Paulos, R. D. & Ramos, J. A. A. (2006). Role of peers in cultural innovation and cultural transmission: evidence from the play of dolphin calves. *International Journal of Comparative Psychology*, 19, 223–40.

Kuhn, T. S. (1962). *The structure of scientific revolutions*. Chicago: University of Chicago Press.

Kummer, H. & Goodall, J. (1985). Conditions of innovative behaviour in primates. *Philosophical Transactions of the Royal Society of London B*, 308, 203–14.

Kyaga, S., Landén, M., Boman, M., Hultman, C. M., Långström, N. & Lichtenstein, P. (2012). Mental illness, suicide and creativity: 40-year prospective total population study. *Journal of Psychiatric Research*, 47, 83–90.

LaBerge, S. P., Nagel, L. E., Dement, W. C. & Zarcone, V. P. (1981). Lucid dreaming verified by volitional communication during REM-sleep. *Perceptual and Motor Skills*, 52, 727–32.

Laland, K. N. & Hoppitt, W. (2003). Do animals have culture? *Evolutionary Anthropology*, 12, 150–9.

Lee, P. C. (1984). Ecological constraints on the social development of vervet monkeys. *Behaviour*, 91, 245–62.

Lefebvre, L., Whittle, P., Lascaris, E. & Finkelstein, A. (1997). Feeding, innovation and forebrain size in birds. *Animal Behaviour*, 53, 549–60.

Lehrer, J. (2012). *Imagine: how creativity works*. Edinburgh: Canongate.

Lieberman, J. N. (1977). *Playfulness: its relationship to imagination and creativity*. New York: Academic Press.

Lillard, A. S., Lerner, M. D., Hopkins, E. J., Dore, R. A., Smith, E. D. & Palmquist, C. M. (2013). The impact of pretend play on children's development: a review of the evidence. *Psychological Bulletin*, 139, 1–34.

Livingston, G. & Levin, R. (1991). The effects of dream length on the relationship between primary process in dreams and creativity. *Dreaming*, 1, 301–9.

Lloyd Morgan, C. (1896). On modification and variation. *Science*, 4, 733–40.

Lorenz, K. (1935). Der Kumpan in der Umwelt des Vogels. *Journal für Ornithologie*, 83, 137–213, 289–413.

Ludwig, A. M. (1990). Alcohol input and creative output. *British Journal of Addiction*, 85, 953–63.

Lyubomirsky, S., King, L. & Diener, E. (2005). The benefits of frequent positive affect: does happiness lead to success? *Psychological Bulletin*, 131, 803–55.

Madden, J. R. (2007). Innovation in sexual display. *Behavioral and Brain Sciences*, 30, 417–18.

Magin, C. M. (1988). *Behavioural development in two species of hyrax living in the Serengeti National Park, Tanzania*. PhD dissertation, University of Cambridge.

Mann, J., Stanton, M. A., Patterson, E. M., Bienenstock, E. J. & Singh, L. O. (2012). Social networks reveal cultural behaviour in tool-using dolphins. *Nature Communications*, 3, 980.

Manning, A. & Dawkins, M. S. (2012). *An introduction to animal behaviour*. Sixth edition. Cambridge: Cambridge University Press.

Marler, P. & Slabberkoorn, H. (2004). *Nature's music: the science of birdsong*. San Diego, CA: Elsevier/Academic Press.

Marten, K., Shariff, K., Psarokos, S. & White, D. J. (1996). Ring bubbles of dolphins. *Scientific American*, August 1996, 83–7.

Martin, P. (1984a). The (four) whys and wherefores of play in cats: a review of functional, evolutionary, developmental and causal issues. In P. K. Smith (Ed.), *Play in animals and humans* (pp. 71–94). Oxford: Blackwell.

Martin, P. (1984b). The time and energy costs of play behaviour in the cat. *Zeitschrift für Tierpsychologie*, 64, 298–312.

Martin, P. (1997). *The sickening mind: brain, behaviour, immunity and disease*. London: HarperCollins.

Martin, P. (2002). *Counting sheep: the science and pleasures of sleep and dreams*. London: HarperCollins.

Martin, P. (2005). *Making happy people: the nature of happiness and its origins in childhood*. London: Fourth Estate.

Martin, P. (2008). *Sex, drugs & chocolate: the science of pleasure*. London: Fourth Estate.

Martin, P. & Bateson, P. (1985). The influence of experimentally manipulating a component of weaning on the development of play in domestic cats. *Animal Behaviour*, 33, 511–18.

Martin, P. & Bateson, P. (2007). *Measuring behaviour: an introductory guide*. 3rd edition. Cambridge: Cambridge University Press.

Martin, P. & Caro, T. M. (1985). On the functions of play and its role in behavioral development. *Advances in the Study of Behavior*, 15, 59–103.

Mason, M. F., Norton, M. I., Van Horn, J. D., Wegner, D. M., Grafton, S. T. & Macrae, C. N. (2007). Wandering minds: the default network and stimulus-independent thought. *Science*, 315, 393–5.

Maurois, A. (1959). *The life of Alexander Fleming, discoverer of penicillin*. London: Jonathan Cape.

McClintock, B. (1950). The origin and behavior of mutable loci in maize. *Proceedings of the National Academy of Sciences*, 36, 344–55.

McGee, P. E. (1979). *Humor: its origin and development*. San Francisco, CA: Freeman.

McGuire, M. T., Raleigh, M. J. & Pollack, D. B. (1994). Personality features in vervet monkeys: the effect of sex age, social status, and group composition. *American Journal of Primatology*, 33, 1–13.

Mckeown, M. (2008). *The truth about innovation*. Harlow, UK: Pearson Prentice-Hall.

McLean, L. D. (2005). Implications for human resource development organizational culture's influence on creativity and innovation: a review of the literature and implications for human resource development. *Advances in Developing Human Resources*, 7, 226–42.

Meaney, M. J. & Stewart, J. (1985). Sex differences in social play: the socialization of sex roles. *Advances in the Study of Behavior*, 15, 1–58.

Mednick, S. A. (1968). The Remote Associates Test. *Journal of Creative Behavior*, 2, 213–14.

Mehta, R. & Zhu, R. (2009). Blue or red? Exploring the effect of color on cognitive task performances. *Science*, 323, 1226–9.

Mendl, M. (1988). The effects of litter-size variation on the development of play-behaviour in the domestic cat: litters of one and two. *Animal Behaviour*, 36, 20–34.

Mendl, M. & Harcourt, R. (1988). Individuality in the domestic cat. In D. C. Turner & P. Bateson (Eds.), *The domestic cat: the biology of its behaviour* (pp. 41–54). Cambridge: Cambridge University Press.

Milteer, R. M. & Ginsburg, K. R. (2012). The importance of play in promoting healthy child development and maintaining strong parent–child bond: focus on children in poverty. *Pediatrics*, 129, e204–e213.

Mitchell, R. W. (2007). Pretense in animals: the continuing relevance of children's pretense. In A. Göncü & S. Gaskins (Eds.), *Play and development: evolutionary, sociocultural and functional perspectives* (pp. 51–75). Hillsdale, NJ: Erlbaum.

Moore, M. & Rudd, S. W. (2008). Follow-up of a pretend play intervention: effects on play, creativity, and emotional processes in children. *Creativity Research Journal*, 20, 427–36.

Morris, D. (1962). *The biology of art: a study of the picture-making behaviour of the great apes and its relationship to human art*. London: Methuen.

Morrison, R. (2004). Informal relationships in the workplace: associations with job satisfaction, organisational commitment and turnover intentions. *New Zealand Journal of Psychology*, 33, 114–28.

Moultrie, J., Nilsson, M., Dissel, M., Haner, U.-E., Janssen, S. & van der Lugt, R. (2007). Innovation spaces: towards a framework for understanding the role of the physical environment in innovation. *Creativity and Innovation Management*, 16, 53–65.

Moyles, J. (2010). Afterword. In J. Moyles (Ed.), *The excellence of play*. 3rd edition (pp. 291–5). Maidenhead, UK: Open University Press.

Mullis, K. (1998). *Dancing naked in the mind field*. London: Vintage Books.

Murdock, M. C. & Ganim, R. M. (1993). Creativity and humor: integration and incongruity. *Journal of Creative Behavior*, 27, 57–70.

Murrin, K. & Martin, P. (2004). *What worries parents: the most common concerns of parents explored and explained*. London: Vermilion.

Nemeth, C. J., Personnaz, B., Personnaz, M. & Goncalo, J. A. (2004). The liberating role of conflict in group creativity: a study in two countries. *European Journal of Social Psychology*, 34, 365–74.

Nettle, D. (2002). *Strong imagination: madness, creativity, and human nature*. Oxford: Oxford University Press.

Nettle, D. (2006). Schizotypy and mental health amongst poets, visual artists, and mathematicians. *Journal of Research in Personality*, 40, 876–90.

Nettle, D. (2007). *Personality: what makes you the way you are?* Oxford: Oxford University Press.

Nettle, D. & Clegg, H. (2006). Schizotypy, creativity and mating success in humans. *Proceedings of the Royal Society B*, 273, 611–15.

Norlander, T. & Gustafson, R. (1998). Effects of alcohol on a divergent figural fluency test during the illumination phase of the creative process. *Creativity Research Journal*, 11, 265–74.

Osborn, H. F. (1896). Ontogenic and phylogenic variation. *Science*, 4, 786–9.

Osborn, A. (1952). *Your creative power: how to use your imagination*. New York: Scribners.

Otto, B. K. (2001). *Fools are everywhere: the court jester around the world*. Chicago: University of Chicago Press.

Paenke, I., Kawecki, T. J. & Sendhoff, B. (2009). The influence of learning on evolution: a mathematical framework. *Artificial Life*, 15, 227–45.

Palmer, S. (2006). *Toxic childhood: how the modern world is damaging our children and what we can do about it*. London: Orion.

Panksepp, J. (1998). *Affective neuroscience*. New York: Oxford University Press.

Panksepp, J. (2007). Neuroevolutionary sources of laughter and social joy: modeling primal human laughter in laboratory rats. *Behavioural Brain Research*, 182, 231–44.

Panksepp, J. (2011). Cross-species affective neuroscience decoding of the primal affective experiences of humans and related animals. *PLoS ONE*, 6, e21236.

Pellegrini, A. D. (1996). *The future of play theory*. Albany, NY: State University of New York Press.

Pellegrini, A. D. (2009). *The role of play in human development*. Oxford: Oxford University Press.

Pellegrini, A. D. (2011). *The Oxford handbook of the development of play*. Oxford: Oxford University Press.

Pellegrini, A. D. & Smith, P. K. (2005). *The nature of play: great apes and humans*. New York: Guilford Press.

Pellis, S. & Pellis, V. (2009). *The playful brain*. Oxford: Oneworld.

Penrose, L. S. & Penrose, R. (1958). Impossible objects: a special type of visual illusion. *British Journal of Psychology*, 49, 31–3.

Piaget, J. (1952). *The origins of intelligence in children*. New York: International Universities Press.

Piaget, J. (1962). *Play, dreams, and imagination in children*. New York: Norton.

Pigliucci, M. & Müller, G. B. (2010). *Evolution: the extended synthesis*. Cambridge, MA: MIT Press.

Plowden, B. (1967). *Children and their primary schools*. London: Central Advisory Council for Education.

POST (2000). *Early years learning*. London: Parliamentary Office of Science and Technology.

Power, T. G. (2000). *Play and exploration in children and animals*. Mahwah, NJ: Erlbaum.

Provine, R. R. (2000). *Laughter: a scientific investigation*. London: Faber & Faber.

Provine, R. R. (2012). *Curious behavior: yawning, laughing, hiccupping, and beyond.* Cambridge, MA: Harvard University Press.

Pruitt, J. N., Burghardt, G. M. & Riechert, S. E. (2012). Non-conceptive sexual behavior in spiders: a form of play associated with body condition, personality type, and male intrasexual selection. *Ethology*, 118, 33–40.

Pruitt, J. N. & Riechert, S. E. (2011). Nonconceptive sexual experience diminishes individuals' latency to mate and increases maternal investment. *Animal Behaviour*, 81, 789–94.

Pryor, K., Haag, R. & O'Reilly, J. (1969). The creative porpoise: training for novel behavior. *Experimental Analysis of Behavior*, 12, 653–61.

Ramachandran, V. S. (1998). The neurology and evolution of humor, laughter, and smiling. *Medical Hypotheses*, 51, 351–4.

Ramsey, G., Bastian, M. L. & van Schaik, C. (2007). Animal innovation defined and operationalized. *Behavioral and Brain Sciences*, 30, 393–437.

Reader, S. M., Hager, Y. & Laland, K. N. (2011). The evolution of primate general and cultural intelligence. *Philosophical Transactions of the Royal Society B*, 366, 1017–27.

Reader, S. M. & Laland, K. N. (2002). Social intelligence, innovation and enhanced brain size in primates. *Proceedings of the National Academy of Sciences USA*, 99, 4436–41.

Reader, S. M. & Laland, K. N. (2003a). *Animal innovation.* Oxford: Oxford University Press.

Reader, S. M. & Laland, K. N. (2003b). Animal innovation: an introduction. In S. M. Reader & K. N. Laland (Eds.), *Animal innovation* (pp. 3–35). Oxford: Oxford University Press.

Reuter, M., Roth, S., Holve, K. & Hennig, J. (2006). Identification of first candidate genes for creativity: a pilot study. *Brain Research*, 1069, 190–7.

Revonsuo, A. (2000). The reinterpretation of dreams: an evolutionary hypothesis of the function of dreaming. *Behavioral and Brain Sciences*, 23, 904–1121.

Root-Bernstein, M. & Root-Bernstein, R. (2006). Imaginary worldplay in childhood and maturity and its impact on adult creativity. *Creativity Research Journal* 18, 403–25.

Root-Bernstein, R. & Root-Bernstein, M. (2001). *Sparks of genius.* Boston, MA: Houghton Mifflin.

Runco, M. A., Millar, G., Acar, S. & Cramond, B. (2010). Torrance tests of creative thinking as predictors of personal and public achievement: a fifty-year follow-up. *Creativity Research Journal*, 22, 361–8.

Runco, M. A., Noble, E. P., Reiter-Palmon, R., Acar, S., Ritchie, T. & Yurkovich, J. M. (2011). The genetic basis of creativity and ideational fluency. *Creativity Research Journal*, 23, 376–80.

Russ, S. W. & Dillon, J. A. (2011). Changes in children's pretend play over two decades. *Creativity Research Journal*, 23, 330–8.

Schredl, M. (1995). Creativity and dream recall. *Journal of Creative Behavior*, 29, 16–24.

Schredl, M. & Erlacher, D. (2007). Self-reported effects of dreams on waking-life creativity: an empirical study. *Journal of Psychology*, 141, 35–46.

Schuldberg, D. (2000). Six subclinical spectrum traits in normal creativity. *Creativity Research Journal*, 13, 5–16.

Scott, G., Leritz, L. E. & Mumford, M. D. (2004). The effectiveness of creativity training: a quantitative review. *Creativity Research Journal*, 16, 361–88.

Scott, S. G. & Bruce, R. A. (1994). Determinants of innovative behavior: a path model of individual innovation in the workplace. *Academy of Management Journal*, 37, 580–607.

Sessa, B. (2008). Is it time to revisit the role of psychedelic drugs in enhancing human creativity? *Journal of Psychopharmacology*, 22, 821–7.

Sharpe, L. L. (2005a). Play fighting does not affect subsequent fighting success in wild meerkats. *Animal Behaviour*, 69, 1023–9.

Sharpe, L. L. (2005b). Play does not enhance social cohesion in a cooperative mammal. *Animal Behaviour*, 70, 551–8.

Sharpe, L. L. (2005c). Frequency of social play does not affect dispersal partnerships in wild meerkats. *Animal Behaviour*, 70, 559–69.

Sharpe, L. L., Clutton-Brock, T. H., Brotherton, P. N. M., Cameron, E. Z. & Cherry, M. I. (2002). Experimental provisioning increases play in free-ranging meerkats. *Animal Behaviour*, 64, 113–21.

Shettleworth, S. J. (2010). *Cognition, evolution and behaviour*. 2nd edition. New York: Oxford University Press.

Sigman, M., Neumann, C., Baksh, M., Bwibo, N. & McDonald, M. A. (1989). Relationship between nutrition and development in Kenyan toddlers. *Journal of Pediatrics*, 115, 357–64.

Simonton, D. K. (1997). Creative productivity: a predictive and explanatory model of career trajectories and landmarks. *Psychological Review*, 104, 66–89.

Simonton, D. K. (2000). Creativity: cognitive, personal, developmental, and social aspects. *American Psychologist*, 55, 151–8.

Simpson, G. G. (1953). The Baldwin effect. *Evolution*, 7, 110–17.

Siviy, S. M., Love, N. J., DeCiccio, B. M., Giordano, S. B. & Seifert, T. L. (2003). The relative playfulness of juvenile Lewis and Fischer-344 rats. *Physiology & Behavior*, 80, 385–94.

Smith, E. F. S. (1991). Early social development in hooded rats (*Rattus norvegicus*): a link between weaning and play. *Animal Behaviour*, 41, 513–24.

Smith, P. K. (1982). Does play matter? Functional and evolutionary aspects of animal and human play. *Behavioral and Brain Sciences*, 5, 139–55.

Smith, P. K. (2010). *Children and play*. Chichester, UK: Wiley-Blackwell.

Smolker, R. J., Richards, A., Connor, R., Mann, J. & Berggren, P. (1997). Sponge carrying by dolphins (Delphinidae, *Tursiops* sp.): a foraging specialization involving tool use? *Ethology*, 103, 454–65.

Sol, D., Duncan, R. P., Blackburn, T. M., Cassey, P. & Lefebvre, L. (2005). Big brains, enhanced cognition, and response of birds to novel environments. *Proceedings of the National Academy of Sciences*, 102, 5460–5.

Spady, T. C. & Ostrander, E. A. (2008). Canine behavioural genetics: pointing out the phenotypes and herding up the genes. *American Journal of Human Genetics*, 82, 10–18.

Spalding, D. A. (1873). Instinct with original observations on young animals. *Macmillan's Magazine*, 27, 282–93.

Spencer, H. (1872). *Principles of psychology*. 2nd edition. New York: Appleton.

Spinka, M., Newberry, R. C. & Bekoff, M. (2001). Mammalian play: training for the unexpected. *Quarterly Review of Biology*, 76, 141–68.

Stamps, J. (1995). Motor learning and the value of familiar space. *American Naturalist*, 146, 41–58.

Sternberg, R. J., O'Hara, L. A. & Lubart, T. I. (1997). Creativity as investment. *California Management Review*, 40, 8–21.

Suslov, I. (1992). Computer model of a 'sense of humour'. I. General algorithm. *Biofizika*, 37, 242 [available at www.arxiv.org/abs/0711.2058v1].

Sutton-Smith, B. (1986). *Toys as culture*. New York: Gardner.

Sutton-Smith, B. (1997). *The ambiguity of play*. Cambridge, MA: Harvard University Press.

Svartberg, K. & Forkman, B. (2002). Personality traits in the domestic dog (*Canis familiaris*). *Applied Animal Behaviour Science*, 79, 133–55.

Sylva, K., Bruner, J. S. & Genova, P. (1976). The role of play in the problem-solving of children 3–5 years old. In J. S. Bruner, A. Jolly & K. Sylva (Eds.), *Play: its role in development and evolution* (pp. 244–57). Harmondsworth, UK: Penguin.

Tan, P. L. & Counsilman, J. J. (1985). The influence of weaning on prey-catching behaviour in kittens. *Zeitschrift für Tierpsychologie*, 70, 148–64.

Teasdale, T. W. & Owen, D. R. (2008). Secular declines in cognitive test scores: a reversal of the Flynn effect. *Intelligence*, 36, 121–6.

Tebbich, S., Sterelny, K. & Teschke, I. (2010). The tale of the finch: adaptive radiation and behavioural flexibility. *Philosophical Transactions of the Royal Society B*, 365, 1099–109.

Tickell, C. (2012). *The early years: foundations for life, health and learning*. London: Her Majesty's Government.

Tinbergen, N. (1963). On aims and methods of ethology. *Zeitschrift für Tierpsychologie*, 20, 410–33.

Torrance, E. P. (1961). Priming creative thinking in the primary grades. *Elementary School Journal*, 62, 139–45.

Torrance, E. P. (1972). Predictive validity of Torrance tests of creative thinking. *Journal of Creative Behavior*, 6, 236–52.

Treadwell, Y. (1970). Humor and creativity. *Psychological Reports*, 26, 55–8.

Trezza, V., Baarendse, P. J. J. & Vanderschuren, L. J. M. J. (2010). The pleasures of play: pharmacological insights into social reward mechanisms. *Trends in Pharmacological Sciences*, 31, 463–9.

Ulrich, R. S. (1984). View through a window may influence recovery from surgery. *Science*, 224, 420–1.

Ulrich, R. S., Berry, L. L., Quan, X. B. & Parish, J. T. (2010). Conceptual framework for the domain of evidence-based design. *HERD: Health Environments Research & Design Journal*, 4, 95–114.

Valentine, G. & McKendrick, J. (1997). Children's outdoor play: exploring parental concerns about children's safety and the changing nature of childhood. *Geoforum*, 28, 219–35.

Van de Castle, R. L. (1994). *Our dreaming mind*. New York: Ballentine.

Vygotsky, L. S. (1967). Play and its role in the mental development of the child. *Soviet Psychology*, 5, 6–18.

Wallas, G. (1926). *The art of thought*. London: Watts.

Ward, H. (2012). All work and no play. *TES Magazine*, 2 November 2012, 5017, 26–30.

Watson, J. (1968). *The double helix: a personal account of the discovery of the structure of DNA*. New York: Scribner.

Wegener, A. (1912). Die Herausbildung der Grossformen der Erdrinde (Kontinente und Ozeane), auf geophysikalischer Grundlage. *Petermanns Geographische Mitteilungen*, 63, 185–95, 253–6, 305–9.

West, M. (1974). Social play in the cat. *American Zoologist*, 14, 427–36.

Whiten, A. & Byrne, R. W. (1988). Tactical deception in primates. *Behavioral & Brain Sciences*, 11, 233–73.

Wiley, D., Ware, C., Bocconcelli, A., Cholewiak, D., Friedlaender, A., Thompson, M., et al. (2011). Underwater components of humpback whale bubble-net feeding behaviour. *Behaviour*, 148, 575–602.

Wood-Gush, D. G. M., Vestergaard, K. & Petersen, H. V. (1990). The significance of motivation and environment in the development of exploration in pigs. *Biology of Behaviour*, 15, 39–52.

Wyles, J. S., Kunkel, J. G. & Wilson, A. C. (1983). Birds, behavior, and anatomical evolution. *Proceedings of the National Academy of Sciences USA*, 80, 4394–7.

Ziv, A. (1989). Using humor to develop creative thinking. *Journal of Children in Contemporary Society*, 20, 99–116.

Index